Food Safety
A Roadmap to Success

Food Safety
A Roadmap to Success

Gary Ades
Ken Leith
Patti Leith

AMSTERDAM • BOSTON • HEIDELBERG • LONDON
NEW YORK • OXFORD • PARIS • SAN DIEGO
SAN FRANCISCO • SINGAPORE • SYDNEY • TOKYO

Academic Press is an imprint of Elsevier

Academic Press is an imprint of Elsevier
125 London Wall, London EC2Y 5AS, UK
525 B Street, Suite 1800, San Diego, CA 92101-4495, USA
50 Hampshire Street, 5th Floor, Cambridge, MA 02139, USA
The Boulevard, Langford Lane, Kidlington, Oxford OX5 1GB, UK

British Library Cataloguing-in-Publication Data
A catalogue record for this book is available from the British Library

Library of Congress Cataloging-in-Publication Data
A catalog record for this book is available from the Library of Congress

ISBN: 978-0-12-811189-5

For information on all Academic Press publications
visit our website at http://www.elsevier.com/

**Working together
to grow libraries in
developing countries**

www.elsevier.com • www.bookaid.org

Publisher: Nikki Levy
Acquisition Editor: Patricia Osborn
Editorial Project Manager: Karen Miller
Production Project Manager: Caroline Johnson
Designer: Ines Cruz

Typeset by MPS Limited, Chennai, India

Dedication

Gary Ades

This book is dedicated to my wife, Lois Ades, for her help in writing and editing the book and for her continuing love and support throughout my career. It is also dedicated to my children, Rebecca and Matthew, and my grandchildren Leo, Alexa, Griffin, Eli, and Sophie, whose food will hopefully be safer because of this book.

Ken Leith and Patti Leith

We dedicate this book to our parents. Fran, Jim, and Dardy—you are missed. Frank—thanks for continuing to encourage us and make us laugh. We thank all of you for your constant focus on showing us the importance of true ethics. You taught us the willingness to do what is right no matter what. Your wisdom helped us realize that even though we know what to do, we still have to convince others to see it, too. It is also dedicated to our children, Nicole and Greg, to whom we have taught the same values. You inspire us to continue to make a difference in the world. Finally, to Lois Ades—many thanks. This book wouldn't be what it is, without your keen eye and patient guidance.

Contents

Section II
Gaining Solid Organizational Commitment

Section III
The Impact of Organizational Structure on Food Safety

Section IV
Implementation—The *Roadmap*

Biography

Gary Ades, PhD, President of G&L Consulting Group, LLC

Gary is President of G&L Consulting Group, LLC. He is a hands-on food professional with over 40 years of experience working in the technical, manufacturing, sales, and marketing areas of the Food and Food Service Industry. He provides Food Safety, Quality Assurance, Crisis Planning, and Strategic Planning assistance to his clients (Farm to Fork) both in the United States and internationally.

Having been a consultant to numerous companies both in the United States and overseas and having had the actual responsibility for Food Safety, Quality, Regulatory Compliance, and R&D (including Product Development) in a wide range of companies, Gary has come to recognize and understand the challenges that Food Safety professionals face in effectively performing their jobs. Many times, it involves understanding how to demonstrate and effectively communicate the value of what they do to others who are involved in the decisions regarding the allocation of resources, whether they are money, people, or departmental cooperation. It can often feel like convincing someone to buy an insurance policy that they do not think they need. He is passionate about sharing his findings and solutions with others to help them succeed and protect their consumers and customers and minimize the risks for their organizations. In order to address these issues, he has conducted numerous workshops and written articles on "Effective Risk Communication to Get Food Safety Resources."

He is also involved in working with academia to understand what would make their curriculums more effective in providing the tools that the Food Safety professionals need to succeed, not the least of which is more business education.

Prior to his current position, he held senior-level positions with Wal-Mart/ Sam's Club, Foster Farms, and Tasty Baking Company, as well as with Arthur D. Little (ADL) and Technomic. He has also been a principal with Marketing Spectrum, a marketing research firm with a significant part of its client base being food and foodservice companies and Technical Food Information Spectrum (TFIS), a leading auditing and food safety consultancy.

Gary is a member of numerous organizations and serves or has served on advisory committees such as the National Advisory Committee on Microbiological Criteria for Foods (NACMCF), the Conference for Food Protection, Food Quality Magazine, Food Safety Magazine, and the Food Safety Summit's Executive Educational Advisory Council. He has served as Secretariat for Safe

Supply of Affordable Foods Everywhere (SSAFE), an international not-for-profit organization, for 6 years.

He received his Bachelor of Science degree and Master of Science degree in Food Science from The Pennsylvania State University and his Doctor of Philosophy degree in Food Science & Technology from Virginia Polytechnic Institute and State University.

Ken Leith, CEO, (e)Gauge, Inc.

Ken is CEO at (e)Gauge, Inc., founded in 2009, providing software services which enable organizations to fully implement strategic initiatives. The software is designed to allow companies to align their resources to ensure achievement of goals. Ken focuses his work on quality, efficiency, and systemic alignment. He is the main architect behind the products for (e)Gauge and Chair of the (e)Gauge Product Development Team, ensuring tools are built to simplify complex challenges by hearing the voice of the customer.

Since 2006, he has also served as a Managing Partner, for (e)Gauge's sister company, EDGES, Inc. His work with EDGES provides a foundation for client companies to realize substantial growth. In addition to effectively leading teams to accomplish business results, he places a strong focus on helping organizations to build metrics, ensuring a productive culture. He has comprehensive experience across his career in the detailed analysis and documentation necessary to create, measure, and enhance efficiency. He is passionate about the integration of technology to support process in order to ensure efficiency. EDGES and (e)Gauge serve industries in logistics, food manufacturing, food handling, and mass retail.

With over 30 years of experience as a leader in business management, customer service, purchasing, quality management, and operations, Ken was previously in an executive-level position over production for a Washington, DC, Division of Brookfield Homes. His experience at Brookfield homes also included Strategic Planning, Process Efficiency, and Purchasing and Operations. During his career he has led the successful conversion of underperforming teams into top producers. He started and led Brookfield's Vendor Quality Council, establishing quality standards with vendor partners to deliver quality homebuilding. In that capacity, he assisted vendor partners in adopting a culture of quality, safety, and collaboration. His team architected and implemented a strategic plan to grow his Division from 400 homes per year to 800 homes per year, ensuring profitable growth while preserving quality.

His corporate career also included time with Ryland Homes and Regency Homes as Director of Customer Service. He has deep experience in media relations. Additionally, he has previously consulted for M/I Homes to build customer service, efficiency, and quality.

He has completed research regarding generational differences in the workplace. He has authored white papers regarding process efficiency, technology integration, strategic planning, and strategic collaboration. He has coauthored guest columns for the NW Arkansas Business Journal and Talk Business Arkansas. He and Patti speak often and are working on their next book collaboration, Think Big; Be Bigger, A Guide to Business Growth.

Patti Leith, CEO, EDGES, Inc.

Since 2001, Patti has been CEO at EDGES, Inc., a services company to help organizations find their potential and exceed their growth goals by fully aligning their resources to achieve those goals. In order to grow, organizations must first develop a short- and long-term plan for growth. They will need to build capacity and efficiency to support that growth. While both are being done, the people doing the work must grow, as well. EDGES' approach includes planning, process efficiency/technology integration, and people development. If an organization wants to grow, it will require a change of direction in its strategic initiatives. After 15 years of working with growth clients, she has found one thing to be profoundly true, without exception: All of the implications of the change in strategic initiatives must permeate the existing culture in order to take hold and become real. Together with Ken, they have led a team to develop methods, tools, and tracking to substantiate culture change.

She also serves as Managing Partner of (e)Gauge, Inc., where she serves on the product development committee. Her predominant focus within the software suite offered by (e)Gauge, Inc. is on the Talent Management modules, which enable organizations to align Job Descriptions with Performance Reviews and KPIs to hold people accountable for their part in a change.

Patti's corporate career spans 16 years with Walmart/Sam's Club, Food Lion Stores, and Sheraton/ITT. She has held corporate leadership positions in Operations, Organizational Development, and Human Resources, with 8 years in senior-level roles.

At SAM's Club, she oversaw the People Development group for SAM's Club's nearly 70,000 employees and managers. While at SAM'S Club, her People Development team won the President's Award for Excellence in 1999. During that same year, her team was recognized by Northwest Arkansas (NOARK)/ SHRM as the most innovative in the field, while she was named SHRM's "Boss of the Year."

She led Human Resources for Food Lion's widespread employees across 1000 stores. Prior to taking this role, she worked in Operations, Succession Planning, and Organizational Development. She was a key member of the committee assembled to respond to ABC's Prime Time Live television expose in 1992, citing Food Lion's Food Safety practices. While Food Lion was able to prove the accusations as staged, the Organizational Development department, under her guidance, implemented state-of-the-art practices in Food Safety.

With an MA in Industrial/Organizational Psychology (and Human Resources Management), and a minor in Statistics and Computer Science, she has authored and validated several skills assessment instruments, including the Inter Face Methods Learning eXcelerator, to foster improved relational influence and build team collaboration and leadership skills. In 2012, she published "Judge Not, A Guide to Influence People Who Think Differently."

Foreword

Food Safety—A Roadmap to Success, by Gary Ades, Ken Leith, and Patti Leith, is truly a path to improving Food Safety in a food business. Food Safety is a discipline and an important profession to protect the public health. The Food Safety professional identifies and manages hazards to prevent human foodborne illnesses and death. The hazards in foods are significant, and continue to show up in new circumstances caused by new pathogens or substances as food processing and food service businesses continue to change; and as new technologies are developed and used by public health agencies to identify sources and causes of the adulteration of food. The Food Safety professional can be found working in academic research, microbiological testing laboratories, government research agencies, environmental health and epidemiology organizations, regulatory agencies, growing, food processing, food service, retail, and distribution businesses. The majority of the knowledge base for the Food Safety professional working in all these organizations comes from college/university-level degree programs in microbiology, quality control, environmental health and epidemiology, food science, and through experience on the job.

Currently, there is no formal training at the college/university level (eg, an undergraduate degree program) that is specific to the implementation and management of the Food Safety discipline in a food business; one that could prepare a Food Safety professional (perhaps like that in environmental health, epidemiology, or microbiology degree programs, for example) to lead Food Safety in a food business. The application of the Food Safety discipline in business has not had, until recently, an advanced-level degree program, like an MBA, to prepare the business manager to lead Food Safety management in a food business. Therefore, the majority of Food Safety professionals in food businesses learn this discipline via bench-marking Food Safety programs in other food businesses, through interaction with other Food Safety professionals in business, participating in trade organizations and science-based organizations, and through important resources like this book written by Food Safety professionals that have successfully implemented and managed the business of Food Safety.

Many Food Safety professionals work to get support and implement Food Safety management programs in a food business atmosphere within their company:

- without buy-in from the business and established budget to support it,
- with no supported value proposition for the value of the program to the business other than speculative cost to the business (eg, lost sales, lower stock prices) "if something goes wrong,"
- with a mandate to only meet minimum regulatory requirements and/or corporate standards observed in other food businesses,
- where support comes only after a Food Safety event that "sheds the light" on current Food Safety management deficiencies within their company.

There are currently several helpful books on the subject matter of Food Safety culture and management in a food business. However, there is currently no resource for the Food Safety professional working in a food business that provides the necessary tested and proven methods to establish a "business model" resource for the Food Safety professional until now.

The authors of this book have actually implemented these business management tools in food and other businesses they have worked in over the course of their very successful business careers. They each are also very active and continue to help others implement these tools as business thought leaders in their current businesses. This book not only serves as a new "how to" resource for carrying out the duties of the Food Safety professional, but the authors are clear that they "want to help the Food Safety professional get the needed resources, that is, people, money, and departmental cooperation, to effectively do their job." Without such resources, of course, Food Safety cannot be properly implemented and sustained in a food business.

This book utilizes the concept of the "puzzle pieces" (culture, organizational commitment and engagement, organizational structure and implementation) along with the "glue" (communication/education/training, metrics to measure success, accountability for change and influence) to hold the pieces together to develop the roadmap for success in implementing a Food Safety program.

The authors provide step-by-step methods and easy-to-use "roadmaps" to implement the principles and requirements of Food Safety culture into a food business. This is not only a book to help Food Safety professionals with their roles, and that which will help a food business establish a Food Safety culture, but it is a book to prevent foodborne illnesses by empowering the food business to manage and prevent them; a true public health innovation.

Hal King
President and CEO, Public Health Innovations LLC
Fayetteville, GA, United States

Introduction:
The Food Safety Puzzle

WHY DID WE WRITE THIS BOOK?

It's funny what can sometimes come out of a casual conversation. While some get drawn into what is wrong with the world and whose fault it may or may not be, others brainstorm ways to change it. Of course, the two are actually related, because the need to make the change is always connected to the description of the problem.

Our team of writers concluded in just such a conversation that the topic of how to actually build a strong Food Safety culture has not been adequately addressed. We decided to share our knowledge and experience with others to provide them with information to impact sustainable culture change and increase commitment to Food Safety. Doing so will provide a solid foundation to enhance the safety of the world's food supply by helping the Food Safety professionals get the resources they need to effectively do their job. All too often, they have responsibility for change, but no direct authority to make it happen. This can lead to frustration and a "Rodney Dangerfield Effect"—or "can't get no respect."

Change is difficult for most people, and most organizations struggle to realize substantial change without great focus and effort. This book will help organizations tackle necessary changes to increase Food Safety. In short, *food organizations will do a better job with Food Safety if they not only know what to do, but also how to do it and why it should be done.* If the deliverables are worth the time and effort, people will actively engage in reaching them.

We decided to write a *guide to assist your organization in the development of strategic initiatives around Food Safety practices and integrate them into your culture to ensure commitment, engagement, and full implementation.* We wanted to write a book that anyone can read and apply within their organization, immediately. Our goal is to offer you methods to adapt proven "best practices" to address the needs of your company from the position you hold.

We want to help the Food Safety professional get the needed resources, that is, people, money, and departmental cooperation, to effectively do their job. We recognize that many times, they have to overcome lack of knowledge, apathy, smugness, false perceptions, and denial by others in the organization. By demonstrating the value (bottom-line impact) of an effective Food Safety program, their job becomes easier. This book will help the Food Safety professional do this and help others connected to this effort support it with their daily actions.

In addition, the food industry needs this book to clearly describe the reasons to consider change and to provide a *Roadmap* of steps and tools to make and sustain the change.

WHY SHOULD YOU READ THIS BOOK?

In this book, you will find detailed *Roadmaps* that will outline steps and tools for you to determine exactly what your company needs and how you can help make that happen, given your position, department, and type of company. Additionally, we will provide you with ways to determine what type of culture your organization has and how you can impact positive change within the cultural dynamics of the organization.

You should read this because it will make the necessary steps for improvement very clear to you and give you tangible tactics to help create a culture that revolves around building key strategies for Food Safety practices. You will benefit from reading this book because the information will help you think about your work differently and give you the tools necessary to help you help your company to succeed. Also, be sure to learn from your mistakes, learn from other's mistakes, and benchmark best practices. There is an interesting quote by George Santayana, philosopher and writer, that is applicable to this situation. "Those who cannot remember the past, are condemned to repeat it."

Basically, most people want to do the right thing, but they aren't sure exactly what to do or how to do it. It is even more difficult to get an entire organization to change. The biggest question is often, "How can I initiate change?", and later, "How can I maintain change?"

WHAT WILL THIS BOOK DO FOR YOU AND YOUR COMPANY?

This book will detail the steps that are necessary to move an organization from one that may only be paying lip service to Food Safety issues, to one that is fully engaged in assuring the right things are being done to protect its customers and consumers, even when nobody is looking. Doing so will *positively impact both the safety and quality of your product, enabling reduced recalls and enhanced customer satisfaction while helping you build market share, increase stakeholder value, and have a positive impact on the company's bottom line.* Additionally, your company's efforts to achieve excellence and maintain Food Safety will *increase your organization's ability to recruit, keep, educate, train, and motivate great people.*

The main goal is to enable your organization to address Food Safety practices as core strategic initiatives. Strategic initiatives are the lifelines that feed the goals, connecting the present to the future. They are the things a company needs to do to change direction and realize growth. They are broad categories of things in which development, improvement, or enhancement are necessary in order for the organization to remain sustainable and competitive.

Often, strategic initiatives focus on "People", "Process," or "Product." As with any strategic initiative, Food Safety should be fully integrated into the organization's day-to-day activities. This book will describe the process by which you can help make this occur.

THE PUZZLE PARTS

We have identified the five main elements needed for effective and positive change. We call this the Food Safety Puzzle.

The Food Safety Puzzle is composed of the five critical pieces needed to make Food Safety a real part of your organization. While they are separate, they are also connected.

They are (see Fig. I.1, The Food Safety Puzzle):

- Culture,
- Organizational Commitment (and Engagement),
- Organizational Structure,
- Food Safety Processes and Procedures,
- Implementation.

Please note that the word puzzle is used as an analogy, not to be confused with an insurmountable task. Puzzles are able to be solved when you have all of the right pieces and fit them together properly. We will use the term "glue" when we discuss how to fit and hold the pieces of the puzzle together.

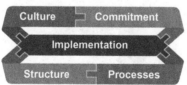

FIGURE I.1   The Food Safety Puzzle.

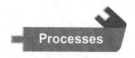

Food Safety Processes and Procedures that are fully implemented and followed are the desired goal of an effective Food Safety program. They are well known and they are an open book test. They are well documented in available manuals and standards. Others have continually reviewed these Food Safety processes and procedures in books, articles, and presentations. They refer to those activities that are developed and implemented to assure Food Safety from farm to fork. These include safe growing, manufacturing/processing, food service operations, retail operations, and distribution. They include Prerequisite Programs, Hazard Analysis Critical Control Point Systems (HACCP), Hazard Analysis Risk-Based Preventive Controls (HARPC), and Continuous Improvement Programs. They make up the Food Safety program and are well defined. For this reason, *this book* will not *introduce or outline the substance of what makes up adequate and effective Food Safety processes and procedures.* Rather, we will focus on the key puzzle pieces involved in making them a reality, every day. The book *will* take a look at some methodologies to change processes from those that don't support Food Safety processes and procedures to processes that offer better compliance. People should not have to prepare for an audit, rather the facilities should always be ready for an audit.

The simple way to summarize most of food safety is:

- Hot food hot,
- Cold food cold,
- Don't cross-contaminate,
- Know who you are buying from,
- Wash your hands.

We will fully explore the other four areas providing you with methods to evaluate each one for your current situation. We will take you through the key issues for each one. We will offer several ways to look at what you need to do within your own organization and within the scope of your role to effect change.

This book will discuss the following four remaining puzzle pieces in four separate sections, even though they are often interrelated.

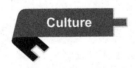

Section I: Developing a Strong Food Safety Culture

This book will discuss the issues that surround culture. What is it? How do you assess it? What elements within a culture support Food Safety as a strategic initiative? Why is it vital to the success of any Food Safety initiative?

We will look at barriers to success and how to overcome them. Then, we will introduce a six-step process which comprises a *Roadmap* for culture change to support Food Safety. Next, we will offer a way to help you determine where your organization's Food Safety culture is today. Finally, we will conclude this section with information regarding what you can do to enhance the Food Safety culture within your organization, from your role.

Culture encompasses what employees believe and what they think they should do. The true litmus test is whether or not employees do the "right thing" when nobody is watching. Culture is talked about in an organization but it is shaped by what is measured and rewarded. It is foundational, because a robust Food Safety culture is critical to making and sustaining the change. Culture is also related to the other puzzle pieces. Cultural change will occur when an organization recognizes, renews, or revitalizes its management commitment to Food Safety. Achieving cultural change is often a byproduct of the implementation of initiatives that improve Food Safety. If a Food Safety initiative positively impacts a company's bottom line, people take notice and are more willing to embrace change. You will want to shape culture to work for you, rather than let it happen on its own.

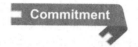

Section II: Gaining Solid Organizational Commitment

We will introduce specific processes to move the entire organization toward the Food Safety goals by demonstrating how to obtain commitment from managers at all levels and their employees. Often, Food Safety programs strive to build Management Commitment, which is not enough. Food handling or processing is usually done by an employee, and overseen by a Manager. Therefore, all levels of employees and their managers must be fully committed.

To be successfully implemented, a strategic initiative must be communicated and well understood. The process of building "owners" (as opposed to "renters") of the initiative at all levels is key to success and will be discussed. This section will also offer methods to influence commitment, and measure the commitment and its impact on targeted results. The concept of building influential communication in order to gain commitment will also be covered fully.

Commitment by its very definition is "the state or quality of being dedicated to a cause or action." Synonyms include words like guarantee, promise, pledge, and responsibility. The implication is that once committed, a person has decided to put forth all of the resources to do what they must to ensure the desired outcome.

Sections I (Culture) and II (Commitment) of this book affect everything. Without a supporting culture and true organizational commitment, your team will not understand how to make the right structural decisions or be successful with their efforts to implement improvement or change. Remember that culture depends on commitment, and commitment will shape culture. They are interdependent.

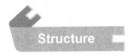

Section III: The Impact of Organizational Structure on Food Safety

Organizational structure is the way an organization is built to get the desired job done. It encompasses who reports to whom (solid line vs dotted line), and also how the work is structured within a position. Organizational structure should be fully aligned with process, that is, the set of steps inherent in getting something done, so that each step within a process is accounted for in a position. Every task within a process should reside in someone's job and be part of his or her Job Description. Process mapping helps to be certain that every step is in someone's Job Description, allowing for more effective implementation.

We will discuss observations regarding the impact of organizational structure on the success of the Food Safety initiatives. This will entail looking at various organizational structures as a means to achieve process objectives. We will specifically discuss ways an organization should look at structure to support Food Safety as a strategic initiative. This section will deal with differences posed by different types of companies. We will provide analysis of advantages and disadvantages for different types of structure. We will also review ways to appropriately update Job Descriptions to enhance and develop necessary skills when changing structure.

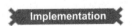

Sections IV: The Food Safety *Roadmap*—A Guide to Implementation

This section will describe a clear *Roadmap* to follow to fully execute the changes. Implementation is the means by which new work is identified, planned, and executed. It involves planning detailed process design/change, and skills development.

Implementation is always done within the context of the organization's strategy. Implementation should encompass desired culture change and plan for it. It will drive structure, because it changes process. Implementation will never happen without full commitment from leaders and those doing the work. This section will explain how to tie together the pieces of the puzzle. This section will review the *Roadmaps* presented thus far and offer a final checklist to follow when implementing change.

All of the puzzle pieces will depend heavily on utilizing the puzzle's "glue" with every puzzle piece.

THE PUZZLE'S "GLUE"

To assure that all of the "puzzle pieces" fit properly and stay together, there are certain activities that form the "glue." We will most often refer to them as the critical ingredients in the "glue." They are involved in and key to every one of the puzzle pieces. They include the following:

- Communication/education/training,
- Metrics to measure success,
- Accountability for change,
- Influence.

Communication/education/training will be addressed in every section, as they are the only tools you have to move, inform, and teach people what will be different. The people in your organization should fully understand the need for the change and the objectives for the change. The prescribed actions must be aligned with the goals for change to be effective. When the change is being discussed and planned, all parties should clearly know what they are trying to impact and why they are trying to impact this particular area. Then, people have to know how to make the change.

Metrics will be addressed in every section, since they are the only way to determine whether your plan is working. Depending on your organization's current commitment to metrics, you may or may not know how you are doing now. It is critical that metrics are identified and measured across the organization, within departments and for each employee. Remember that measurement drives behavior, so don't measure anything that doesn't tell you how you are doing, compared with your goal.

Accountability will be addressed in every section as well, because the leaders/managers need to address when people are not implementing the change. This is a key means of making sure that the right things are taking place to fully realize your goals. Most often, good accountability cannot exist without communication/education/training, or without metrics.

Influence is the art of changing the way a person thinks. Every puzzle piece requires a high level of influence and methods to do so will be described in all four sections. The goal of influence is to convince people to change their behavior. Sometimes influence can include persuasion which also enables people to change their mind about something.

Mission and vision are a good place to start to communicate and affect change, but they only begin to define the targeted shifts needed in culture.

Simply saying you will do it or that you are committed to it does not mean that individuals will change. Without a comprehensive plan for measurement and accountability, the Mission and Vision statement are just words. You have to tell people what you are going to do, tell them why, show them how to do it, provide them with the necessary resources to do it, and make sure they do it.

As you can see, there are a lot of moving parts. This may be complex, but it is doable. In order to help you understand the pieces of the puzzle, the sections and their chapters will define the bigger picture and the desired end-state for the target, along with illustrative examples. The chapters will discuss the barriers to achieving the desired end-state, and present solutions and methodologies. The reader will learn how to attain the target and apply the concepts to their situation.

Most chapters will offer suggestions about what you can do to impact change, questions you can ask, dialog you can prompt, and things you can do to move the organization closer to fully embracing Food Safety.

Why Keep Reading?

To learn how to get an effective Food Safety program implemented and maintained in your company. When an organization proactively decides to make a firm commitment to Food Safety, it is similar to purchasing an insurance policy, in that it protects against catastrophe. Some companies, however, refuse to change focus and do not make the decision to commit time, resources, and departmental cooperation to the improvement of their Food Safety system until they experience the crippling emotional and monetary cost of a mistake. By then, it is likely too late.

Tangible results of your team's changes in the Food Safety culture will positively impact quality, customer and consumer satisfaction, and the company's bottom line. Additionally, you will enable your organization to effectively recruit and keep stronger people, because people want to be a part of something great.

The book will help you and your company succeed and prosper. It will provide you with tools to execute ideas that will support and grow Food Safety within your organization. The book, itself, can also be used as a valuable tool and resource when communicating with all levels within your organization.

Section I

Developing a Strong Food Safety Culture

Chapter 1

What Is an *Effective* Food Safety Culture?

Chapter Outline

WHAT IS CULTURE? THE BIG PICTURE

In order to manage culture, you must first understand it. In short, it is "What happens when nobody is looking." Culture is solely shaped by "What's rewarded around here?"

That being said, many things create and shape culture, including history, experience, norms, fears, goals, and dreams. Culture is both fragile and strong at the same time. It can change without warning. It can be influenced by change in the organization and by things your team experiences, such as changes in strategic direction or organizational structure or ownership. It is greatly impacted by mergers, acquisitions, and advances in technology. Culture can provide a strong, solid guide for everyone's actions and how they should be delivered. It can be shaped to work for you by rewarding the behavior that you want.

Culture is patterned after what people talk about, but it is shaped by what is measured and rewarded. Positive change happens when you tell people what will be different, measure the things you are trying to change and hold people accountable for their part in

Food Safety. DOI: http://dx.doi.org/10.1016/B978-0-12-811189-5.00001-5

achieving results. If an employee who does excellent work gets recognized, rewarded, or promoted, the message is that excellence matters. But if someone is recognized, rewarded, or promoted who has been allowed to take shortcuts, the message is that excellence is not important. The culture begins to accept mediocrity. If allowed to continue, the message can encourage careless risk-taking and noncompliance.

HOW IS CULTURE CHANGED? THE METHODOLOGY

Proactively, your team of top leaders and managers can make a planned culture shift to support the company's goals. In order to do that, your leadership team has to plan for the change, but all managers have to be made aware of what is happening and be ready to respond.

Think about playing a game. The game is played according to established and known rules. They are explained up front to the players. In most games, points are accumulated when players score. In organized games, there is usually a referee to be sure people are following the rules and a coach to help people play more effectively. In most games, the scores enable the win.

With culture, you must set the rules of the game to be played the way you want it to be played. These are *established expectations* that must be communicated to all members of your organization. They should be told what to do, why they are being asked to do it and be given specific instructions as to how it should be done. This will likely include education and training.

Goals must then be established that are linked to incentives. This is the way that scores will be kept. The plan should incent, reward, and recognize players to achieve the goals. Remember, scores enable the win, and in an organization, goal achievements should be recognized. Incentives/rewards can be tangible, such as raises to base compensation, bonuses, and other financial rewards. They can also include promotions, recognition awards, prizes, or perks. Incentives/rewards can also be intangible, such as better job satisfaction, less confusion, and making their jobs easier. Whatever the reward, it should guide behavior to meet the goals. The people making the change should be very clear on what behavior is desired. Metrics come into play here, as that is how an organization keeps score. When culture is linked to metrics, people do more of what is rewarded and less of what is not.

Now, let's look at the game personnel responsibilities. The referee is the one who points out when a person is not playing by the rules. This is a function of leadership and should be done by everyone in your organization who manages others. The coach is the one who helps players get better. This is also a function of leadership and everyone with responsibility over another person should be tasked with helping them play better in the new environment.

In short, the "game" must be set up to be played the right way, allowing "players" to understand and meet expectations in order to ensure that culture is actually enhanced at the same time. This allows the organization to embrace the change.

WHAT IS AN EFFECTIVE FOOD SAFETY CULTURE? THE DESIRED END STATE

There is that question again... Probably, one of the main reasons you are reading this book. Characteristics of an effective Food Safety culture include (but are not limited to) the following characteristics.

- Food Safety is everyone's goal not just a specific group in a company.
- Decisions are easily made where Food Safety is concerned, and all employees are committed to Food Safety.
- Departments work together to determine and make the right decisions.
- Teams work on problems together.
- Excellence is measured and rewarded.
- Food Safety is not compromised for the sake of meeting budgets.
- Noncompliance has consequences.
- Everyone does the right thing, even when nobody is looking.
- People talk about Food Safety, often and in detail.
- People don't take shortcuts, even when they are tired or stressed.
- Workers take pride in their work.

- Decisions are made according to clearly defined directions or objectives.
- People care about excellence.
- People always want to make things just a little bit better.
- Technology supports effective task completion.
- Food Safety is always considered and talked about when decisions are made.

Instilling a culture of excellence can create a highly engaged workforce. Leadership teams should pursue total organizational commitment through intentional cultural change.

Full transition must be supported by effective communication, education, training, metrics to measure the change, and unflappable accountability to reward success and address needs for improvement.

A CASE STUDY—WHAT IS MISSING?

This case study is based on some combination of things the authors have seen in their work with organizations. Some of the variables and characteristics were changed to ensure full anonymity. Read through these with an analytical eye to see if you can spot the key elements that led to the challenge or the success outlined in the case study. Look for the learning opportunities that might be applicable to your situation now, or in the future.

Company A: Medium Sized, Food Production

The leadership team in this company worked together and developed a strong commitment to fully embrace Food Safety. They strongly believed they were headed in the proper direction and were committed to proactively structuring operations to ensure change before any problems surfaced. They collaboratively began to embrace a shift in the way they thought about production from "fast and cheap" to "good and reliable." They were certain it would lead to better customer perception, increased revenues, and the ability to attract and retain the best talent in the industry. They talked about it often and offered education about why it was important, and training on how to do it. Customer perception began to improve.

Everyone got busy as this went along, so they didn't do everything necessary. Nevertheless, progress was visible, which increased engagement. The CEO talked often about the initiatives and their importance.

Then, one day, the CEO left the company to run a bigger company. Within 1 month of his departure, people stopped talking about Food Safety as much as they had been. Teams get far less productive when major change occurs. A change of this nature can paralyze some people. Slowly, they began to lose focus. As a result, they began to see more returns of their products.

Not long after, a new CEO was appointed from outside of the company. She came in and immediately linked goals to building revenue and increasing margins. She cut back on some of the programs still in place, due to cost. This led to increased turnover, lower quality, and dropping revenues in the subsequent 18 months.

This classic culture failure (the inability to fully shift culture to support strategic change) occurred for two major reasons. The first and most obvious reason was a lack of commitment from the new CEO. There was another component, however, because the decline started before she arrived. It began to quickly decline as soon as the first CEO left. Why?

Remember *"Full transition must be supported by effective communication, education, training, metrics to measure the change, and unflappable accountability to reward success and address needs for improvement."*

Prior to the first CEO's departure, they had built commitment through communication, education, and training. They recognized progress. So, the missing part was the accountability, backed by the metrics to measure the change. If they had put all the necessary parts in place so that the system was set for success, it would not have unraveled so quickly. Managers would have kept looking at indicators and adjusting behaviors where needed. Leaders would have kept asking questions to be sure implementation was occurring as planned. Engagement would have been greater.

One critical piece of gaining success is to have all systems in place to minimize risk and make it very difficult for them to be overridden by what is perceived as production necessity, which in most cases is *"get to market as quickly and as cheaply as possible."*

This prevailing mentality can create a significant culture failure, because it indirectly sets the expectation that shortcuts are acceptable and necessary.

WHAT CAN YOU DO, NOW?

As this section progresses, you will be provided with tools to understand the type of culture you currently have and how you, in your role, can enhance it to more deeply embrace the goals you have for Food Safety, thus laying a foundation for better commitment. For now, think about the current situation in your organization.

Here are some questions to consider...

1. What are the key drivers for your present culture?
2. What are the advantages of your present culture?
3. What are the challenges of your present culture?
4. How might you enhance or change your culture to increase the organizational commitment to Food Safety?

Then, start talking about it to others. Ask for their input; get them thinking; build ideas together.

Chapter 2

What Gets in the Way?
Barriers and Solutions

Chapter Outline

YOUR MOST COMMON BARRIERS

Now that we know what culture is, how to shape it and the characteristics of an effective Food Safety culture, let's look at the main reasons organizations fail to truly commit to the actions that support solid Food Safety practices. We will introduce and explore the most common barriers, define their challenges and offer solutions.

The biggest barriers to changing an organization's commitment to Food Safety are:

- *Skepticism/engagement*
  - Change resistance
    - Historical perspective does not suggest a need for change
    - Perception that this would affect the organization's ability to be cost-competitive

Food Safety. DOI: http://dx.doi.org/10.1016/B978-0-12-811189-5.00002-7

- *Degree of experience and/or knowledge of decision makers and influencers*
  - Leaders
  - Employees
- *Degree of leadership commitment*
  - Absent
  - Weak
  - Not defined
- *Not being integrated into the overall strategy*
  - Not strategic
  - Not seen as "must have"
  - Viewed as "overhead"
- *Resources*
  - People
  - Money
  - Time
  - Departmental cooperation
  - Goals
    - Agreement with goals
- *Communication about the need for change is inadequate*
  - Process
  - Roles and expectations
  - Accountability measures (appropriate metrics).

Now let's look at each of these barriers, their challenges and some possible solutions.

BARRIERS, CHALLENGES, AND SOLUTIONS

As you become more familiar with the barriers, take a look at whether or not they are present in your organization. Determine whether or not the solutions, or some variation of them, could work in your situation. Most importantly.... start a dialogue and get people talking. If these solutions don't fit your needs exactly, you and the people you work with should be able to come up with some alternatives based on the information included in this chapter.

Skepticism/Engagement

Overcoming skepticism and historical behavior at management levels can often be a problem. Often-heard comments that demonstrate this skepticism or resistance are: "We've never had a problem before"; "It's too expensive"; "It's not worth the money"; "I'll take the chance"; "No one else is doing this"; "It will put us at an economic disadvantage"; and/or "That's overkill." It is not enough for an organization to say they are doing something differently. They must convince everyone in the organization that there is a need for the change and that they are serious about making the changes. Even if they are doing everything they should to implement that change, there is the possibility that people will not embrace it because they think the change won't really happen.

- *Challenge*: People resist change unless they can see the benefit.
- *Challenge*: Past efforts to change have not been successful.
- *Solutions*—This should be addressed in the communication plan. It will take time to convince people. The best way to make headway quickly in this area is to clearly describe the need, clearly describe the change and how it will affect them and then measure and hold people accountable. There is no better way to make a lack of engagement unacceptable than to simply not allow it. If you see that the employees and/or the managers are not following the commitment, make someone aware. If you are in a management or leadership position, ask enough questions to be sure people are moving from a "renter to an owner mentality" for their part of the Food Safety process.

Degree of Experience and/or Knowledge of Decision Makers and Influencers

If leaders have never experienced a Food Safety situation they tend to think that it will never happen to them. Also, when an organization does not know what to do, they are far less likely to do it. This may preclude any real emphasis on the issue, just by the very nature that people tend to put off doing things they aren't sure how to do.

- *Challenge*: Convincing leaders that Food Safety problems can happen to their company.
- *Challenge*: Leaders don't know what to do or how to do it, so they don't try.
- *Challenge*: Leaders try, but employees don't know how the change will impact what they do.
- *Challenge*: Employees try but they haven't learned enough about it to make the right decisions.
- *Solutions*—Describe the need for Food Safety in terms that leaders will understand. Communicate often and extensively about the need. Educate often and extensively on the why—the reason to do it. Train employees on how the process is required to occur. To do so, effectively, someone in the organization must develop an effective communication plan.

Degree of Leadership Commitment

When there is not a visibly strong leadership commitment, the organization simply will not commit. Likely, the absence of this commitment leads to many other barriers that are not identified or addressed. The reality is that nothing else can get changed without better commitment from the leadership team. This is a main theme in the culture types discussed in Chapter 4 "What Can You Do? Your Role and Its Impact on Positive Culture Change." When leadership commitment is absent or only haphazardly put forth, it is likely that very little will change in culture.

- *Challenge*: Leaders don't talk about the need to change and don't commit. The issue is absent from company discussions and from company meetings.
- *Challenge*: Leaders pay lip service to the need to change and commit, but don't actually change anything. The commitment is weak because it is not backed up with solid activities.
- *Solutions*—Leaders should be shown appropriate information often enough to get them to understand the need for a stronger commitment. Books, articles, forums, and case studies can help. Don't make the communication overly technical. Communicate facts and their implications to the company.

Relating implications to the "bottom line" is a very effective communication too. Frequent contact with peers who have made this commitment can also help. If you are reading this and not in a leadership position, you can encourage and influence others by providing information to present to management. If you are reading this and you are in a leadership position and know your leadership team isn't fully committed, reach out to peers to help you and the other members of your team. The realization that doing so is not only insurance against catastrophe, but also the key to offering the safest product and getting and keeping not only customers but the best employees.

Not Being Integrated Into the Overall Strategy

Failure to integrate Food Safety Initiatives into the organization's strategy will quickly disconnect the commitment from the practices. When an organization makes a commitment to Food Safety and adjusts their practices, structure and culture to support it, it must be integrated into a core business strategy for this commitment and investment to work.

- *Challenge*: Food Safety is said to be a strategic initiative, but it is not talked about in strategic planning meetings. Therefore, commitment to it will very likely not be made or will diminish over time.
- *Challenge*: Food Safety is seen as a "should have," not as a strategic, "must have" need. This makes leaders feel like they have to do it, rather than wanting to do it. Again, this will diminish the commitment and ultimately waste valuable resources.
- *Solutions*—Influence a change in mindset so that Food Safety is embraced because it protects the organization. Add Food Safety as a strategic initiative to your overall strategic plan. You can also enhance the definition of your quality initiatives to encompass the full scope of Food Safety. Good Food Safety usually has a positive impact on quality. Connecting Food Safety to the company's strategy signifies that it is an important component to long-term success. Immediately begin to link all Food Safety activities and projects to its corresponding strategy.

Resources

This is a major barrier, due to its breadth. Many do not embrace Food Safety initiatives because of lack of resources. This is most often because resources cost money in one way or another. Thus, the reason for this barrier may really be a hesitancy to invest or spend extra money. There are several implications (challenges) within this.

- *Challenge*: First of all, for Food Safety initiatives to be put in place, it requires the organization to have an organizational structure of people to support it. This may mean an immediate increase in head count, salaries, and benefits, since these people are usually added to focus on the Food Safety initiatives. In some situations, the responsibilities might actually go to other people in the organization. This approach is not ideal, if it just adds responsibility to an already overburdened employee and therefore minimizes the effectiveness of the person to do this new job as well as their original job. We believe that someone must have the full-time responsibility and authority for Food Safety. The organizational structure options and their implications will be explored fully in Section III—The Impact of Organizational Structure on Food Safety.
- *Challenge*: Next, even if the organization commits to adding people, or simply adds duties to existing people, doing the right things takes time and time translates to money. Additional time is often needed to complete the task effectively. This may result in lower productivity. Time is needed to educate and train people to complete the task effectively. This includes training managers. Time is needed on the part of the managers to check that the task is being done correctly. Finally, time is needed to address discrepancies. Operational goals are usually based on getting things out the door as quickly as possible for as little expense as possible. Fast and cheap leads to better profits. Or does it?
- *Challenge*: Goals are generally set with stringent financial objectives in mind and may not encourage leaders to do the right things, because there are consequences for not meeting these goals.

- *Solutions*—If the reason for not implementing an effective Food Safety program is financially based, then the solution rests with the ability of the leadership team to *develop and believe in a strong business case for the expenditures.* The case should be based on the premise that this is insurance, and should understand the consequences of not committing resources if things go wrong. The case should also address the market value of the changes inherent in doing things correctly. This includes better quality, better consumer satisfaction, increased market share, better customer satisfaction, and greater retention of employees because of increased job satisfaction.
  - Goals must be adjusted to reflect realistic financial numbers that will occur when the right thing is continuously done.
  - Once done, the organization will need to:
    - Provide solid process definition
    - Develop clear expectations including appropriate metrics to measure performance
    - Outline role expectations
    - Educate and teach people how to do the right thing
    - Teach managers how to effectively manage so that people do the right thing.

Communication About the Need for Change Is Inadequate

Often, change occurs in an organization without an adequate and effective communication plan. Someone in the organization needs to take ownership and lead this plan or the organization should seek support from an outside agency to commit the resources for proper communication. When the communication is not done well, the organization will never fully understand the intended changes, their intended benefits or the consequences if they are not addressed.

- *Challenge*: The process is missing information. Once the commitment is made and people learn the information necessary to change the process, they may do so in a vacuum without involving others in that change. As a result, the change will become final without input from all of the parties involved.

Therefore, key points will be missed and make implementation at all levels difficult.

- *Challenge*: Expectations and roles are unclear. People don't know what to do or how the change impacts them. The message that the organization is changing focus may not be strong enough to get people to make the change. People need to understand why change is needed, as well as how the company will benefit from the change and how they will be affected. Each person required to do something differently should have the appropriate education and training about what they should be doing differently.
- *Challenge*: Accountability measures are not connected, clearly communicated and/or managed.
- *Solutions—(note that all are needed and this will be dealt with in greater detail in Section IV—Implementation—The Roadmap)*
  - o Map the process with input from all of those who are involved in the process.
  - o Verify the process.
  - o Finalize the process and develop documentation.
  - o Identify all positions impacted; develop education and training.
  - o Develop a leadership education and training plan for all affected, based on their knowledge. Involve them wherever possible in the previous steps.
  - o Develop a communication plan, highlighting the commitment as a focal point.

REMEMBER...

Start dialogue and get people talking. If these solutions don't exactly mirror your needs, you and the people you work with should work together to come up with some alternatives.

Chapter 3

How Does Culture Come to Be?
A *Roadmap*

Chapter Outline

TWO METHODS OF CULTURE DEVELOPMENT

When an organization decides to embrace something as a strategic initiative, there is a need to change behavior in the organization for this change to happen. If an organization wants the change to be substantial and become fully rooted in the workplace so employees do the right thing even when nobody is looking, they will only do so through a shift in culture.

There are generally two ways a culture comes to be. Let's take a look at the two possibilities.

1. *Culture can happen on its own.* This occurs when leaders do nothing to proactively define what culture should be for the changes to take root, and then they don't communicate expectations, institute metrics or set up any reward to support desired change.

   This is not ideal because an organic culture that evolves on its own, usually contains elements that are not conducive to what the organization is trying to accomplish. When culture happens on its own, people look to communication, rewards

Food Safety. DOI: http://dx.doi.org/10.1016/B978-0-12-811189-5.00003-9
17

and measures already in place to determine what is important. If the leadership team hasn't re-defined these, they will almost certainly continue to shape the undesirable elements within the culture that led to the need for the changes in the first place.

In the absence of good leadership planning around culture, mediocrity, frustration, fear, and lack of trust with leadership decisions can develop in the workforce. Additionally, if the leaders talk about needed change but do not do the things to enhance culture, this may lead to skepticism. The result is a scenario in which the organization has "renters," rather than "owners." They will wait to be told to do the right thing, rather than make it their daily practice to do the right thing. Negative aspects to culture are the biggest barriers to full engagement of the workforce.

One indicator that your culture may have undesirable characteristics is if your employee turnover rate is high. Another is if you have trouble attracting a high-quality workforce. If either of these pertains to you, think of ways to impact your organization to understand that shaping culture is critical. It is never too late to start.

2. *Culture can be planned and shaped by leadership to support the organization's direction.* This occurs when the leaders work to proactively define what culture should be for the changes to take root, and then they define and communicate expectations, initiate metrics and set up rewards to support desired change.

This is ideal because it leaves less to chance. It adjusts things in the organization to ensure the desired behaviors are known and executed. This type of culture has better employee engagement. The most important ingredients in shaping this are the communication of expectations, the identification of metrics, and a management team that holds others accountable. In doing this, the entire leadership team will rely on their ability to influence others around them to make the necessary changes. Remember, these elements are the "glue" in the Food Safety Puzzle. They will require collaborative effort to align efforts to shape the culture.

Food Safety and its related activities and goals will not only lead to safe food, but also to quality enhancements. This will impact the consumer's health (always expected) and their satisfaction with your product/service (the differentiator in their choice of brand). Food Safety is foundational to any organization that deals with food, and it should be fully integrated into existing strategic business goals and worked into culture. If your organization's goals do not include Food Safety, your team should quickly begin dialog to develop specific goals with respect to Food Safety. Be certain that Food Safety is one of your key strategic initiatives. Don't put it under Customer Service, or Process Efficiency, as it will not get the attention it deserves.

ROADMAP: STEPS TO PLANNED CULTURE CHANGE

In order to design and shape culture that supports your organization's goals, there is an easy, six-step program for your team to follow. This process, however, assumes that everyone in the organization has the same goal and will commit the time and resources necessary to make it happen. We realize that is not always the case.

If you feel your organization is lacking true commitment, read these steps anyway. They are your desired end state to shape culture. In Section II – Gaining Solid Organizational Commitment, we will take a look at ways to increase commitment through directly influencing your team about the needs.

The steps listed below comprise the *Roadmap* that can guide you on your journey to influence and move your team towards recognizing the need for change.

1. *Plan: Integrate Food Safety into your strategic initiatives/ goals*—If your organization regularly plans, re-direct the agenda to encompass discussion about Food Safety. If your organization does not regularly plan, influence the leadership team to set aside time for planning. As mentioned previously, the full integration of Food Safety into your organization begins when leaders decide to come together in a collaborative effort to set strategic business goals and determine what is important to building a sustainable future. *Food Safety should be prominent on your organization's list of strategic business goals.*

    a. Without goals, there is no target.

    b. Without collaboration, there is little commitment to the goals.

    c. Without planning, there is not a clear path to achieve goals.

    d. Including Food Safety prominently in your organization's goal set is the best first step to make change happen.

2. *Dialog: Get people talking about Food Safety; make it top of the mind*—When leaders talk about Food Safety across the organization, with each other and with the teams they lead, it sends a strong message that Food Safety is serious and important. Remember that communication is a critical ingredient in the "glue" necessary to be successful. While there are many different layers to successful communication during change efforts, it starts with talking about what you are trying to do.

    a. During initial and subsequent discussions, leaders should maintain an ongoing dialog about issues surrounding the question "What kind of company do we need to be, to be able to fully embrace Food Safety?"

    b. Your team's goal is to develop a culture where everyone follows the required steps to ensure safe food, even when nobody is watching. Speak about this often.

    c. Food Safety must be top of the mind, every day.

3. *Change Process: Figure out what needs to change to bridge the gap between where you are and what you are trying to accomplish*—Identify the processes that will support the changes you are trying to accomplish. Consider the company's history and what is happening today. Outline the desired workflow with a high enough level of detail to help others follow the steps necessary for change to occur.

4. *Communicate Change: Make sure everyone knows what to do, why they are doing it and how to complete it the correct way.*

    a. The changing of the culture will begin when your organization tells people it is changing (Communication), why it is changing (Education) and shows them how to make the changes (Training).

    b. Any change must be supported with teaching, which is made up of education and training.

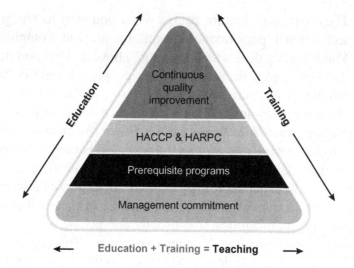

Education + Training = **Teaching**

Effective communications systems include messages that are:
- Understandable
- Tangible
- Compelling
- Rapid
- Relevant
- Reliable
- Repeated
- Multilingual
- Culturally sensitive.

5. *Develop Success Measures: Set the stage for the game to be played correctly*—Determine how you will measure compliance and commitment. Measurement is another important "glue" ingredient. Without it, it is very difficult to measure progress and impossible to change culture. Culture is simply—what is measured around here...? Measures will help answer questions. How will you know the right things are happening? How will you know positive change towards your goals is occurring? The most obvious answer is to reward people for following process. Often, a financial person or committee will take over that work to be sure that measures are meaningful, accurate, and well understood by those who are making decisions.

    a. The shaping of culture begins when you start to recognize and reward performance, commitment, and compliance. Make it a big deal when people go above and beyond doing the right thing. Be sure that only people who are embracing the changes are rewarded. Culture will slip backwards if someone is rewarded for noncompliance or taking short cuts.

6. *Implement and Hold Accountable: Begin the culture change when you change and monitor process*—It is best to empower one central key person in the organization to identify the best way to facilitate a plan to shape culture. In larger organizations, this may be a team of people or a committee in charge of culture. In smaller organizations, it is usually one person who is really good at communicating direction to everyone. This is part of the planning process and done in tandem with the change efforts.

    a. Hold people accountable: Managers must deal with noncompliance consistently and hold people accountable for their actions. Accountability starts with the act of a manager focusing on performance. Often, leadership development programs can provide a foundation for managers to be able to do this well.

        i. Managers should observe if someone is not changing in the way they were asked and taught to do; if they are not doing something that the process requires; or if they are doing it wrong.

        ii. The next step is to guide the person to the right behavior with specific and direct, yet diplomatic, language. Think of this as the "walk with me" or the "let me show you how" conversation. This does not have to become a disciplinary conversation or one in which the employee feels they are in big trouble.

            o While disciplinary conversations may be needed at times, the use of the word accountability does not mean "pin them to the wall for non-performance." Rather it means, notice, assist, guide, and coach. Provide a mixture of encouragement and enforcement. Give them a chance to do the right things. Then, if they don't, appropriate action can be taken.

- ○ If noncompliance has been accepted for some time, start from the beginning with a discussion. Since the situation cannot continue to persist, it may move to a disciplinary process more quickly. When someone is not committing to the needed change a deadline for compliance must be set.
- ○ There are some noncompliance activities that are egregious and warrant immediate discipline and dismissal. Educate managers as to what those are. Provide tips to spot problems and provide a formal process to deal with them.

If your organization has previously implemented change but did not shift culture to support the work, people may not be following new processes. You will want to check and adjust the "glue" ingredients, even though the process work is in motion. Failure to embrace can almost always be tied back to challenges in communicating, measuring, or holding others accountable. Provide the incentives and resources necessary to succeed. Show respect and reinforce the correct, shared values and beliefs in the culture with new and current employees.

MAKE SURE EVERYTHING SUPPORTS CHANGE...

One of the best examples we have seen of an organization that failed to implement culture change properly was an agricultural organization beginning to export to Latin America. The decision to export was made quickly and without planning. The change was reviewed by two key people in charge of shipping, but no measures of the process were put into place.

The export process required a high level of expertise in freight forwarding. The company needed to receive the shipments quickly and the United States had to deal with timely border crossings. Employee training and planning would ensure product safety and cut back on shipments being held at the border for technicalities in the country's freight forwarding guidelines. The company skipped that part. The organization began seeing a sharp increase in demands for consumer refunds due to late product arrival. This also lengthened the supply chain and the customer's ability to utilize the product as needed.

It took a while for the US company to notice the problem because the international claims were measured with the domestic claims. Since this was a new business, the percent of business was not enough to make a noticeable change in the claim numbers. An astute sales manager noticed that a lot of shipments were being held up. He began to look at claims for the international business separately. Alarmed at what he found, he began to assess its impact on profit.

He took those numbers to the leadership team and asked for assistance in the form of a planning session, focused on process. The team set aside two days to plan ways to minimize the impact that lack of process was having on their profit. During their discussions, they realized they weren't measuring nearly enough to determine whether shipments were being handled correctly. During the 2 days the team was working together, they received notice that two shipments with the same shipping coordinator's signature were being held at the border. Further inspection showed that this had happened several times in the past, as well. Her supervisor left the planning meeting to address the infractions with her.

The company had a rewards program in place to recognize high-level performance by employees. These rewards were based on service/support to either customers or fellow employees. One week after the infractions, the shipping coordinator won a very visible award for excellent performance. This sent a strong message to her co-workers that mistakes are okay and friendly behavior is more important than accurate work.

A multiple-tiered rewards program was set in motion a few months later, after lengthy process efficiency work. All of this could have been proactively averted up front with planning of process, change communication, and accurate progress measurement that is aligned to recognition and rewards.

WHAT IF...

Now, what happens if the perfect environment does not exist for people to do this? What if people don't see the need to focus on always doing the right thing? What if your teams don't plan together? What if goals are supporting actions that aren't consistent with what you are trying to accomplish? What if your organization doesn't communicate change well? What if you don't measure things? What if your managers can't hold people accountable? If any of these situations exist, you have your work cut out for you. You can be successful if you keep your goal in mind and gather the moving pieces to support them. Planning for change is the key.

As you read this book, we will often describe different types of plans. This chapter introduced ways to create a Strategic/Business Goals Plan that drives everything. In this chapter, we also advocate several plans to support the implementation of the Strategic/Business Goals Plan. These include a *Culture Change Plan*, a *Change Communication Plan*, a *Measurement Plan*, and an *Accountability Plan*. These different pieces are all a part of the master Strategic/Business Goals Plan. These are the keys to the Food Safety Puzzle.

We will continue to deal with change in the form of a plan as we go deeper into the content. Remember that any plan, regardless of the type of plan it is or what it is trying to accomplish is simply that... a plan. Plans change and the owners of the plans must be aware of changing needs and be flexible enough to change it. Think of a pilot who files a flight plan. That is what he/she thinks they will do when they are on the ground. Then, they get up in the air. Things change and the plan needs to be modified quickly. Their safety depends on their ability to spot the need to adjust and to adjust it immediately. Be a pilot within your organization.

In the next chapter, we will discuss what you can do to change culture, based on the scope of your role and the type of culture you are experiencing.

Chapter 4

What Can You Do? Your Role and Its Impact on Positive Culture Change

Chapter Outline

Let's review the content thus far. The Introduction offered an overview of the book itself, and the previous chapters, thus far, have outlined the following:

- Chapter 1 "What Is an Effective Food Safety Culture?" explored what culture actually is and *how* you can change it. It outlined a comprehensive *list of things you would see in the desired situation* upon being successful at getting the change to occur.
- Chapter 2 "What Gets in the Way? Barriers and Solutions" explored the many *barriers* to the culture change and offered *solutions* to overcome them. While these may not exactly match your situation, many ideas for change can be applied to your situation.
- Chapter 3 "How Does Culture Come to Be? A *Roadmap*" discussed the importance of managing culture change, rather than letting it happen randomly. This chapter outlined six steps in a process to change culture, which is the Roadmap to *intentionally shift culture.*

Food Safety. DOI: http://dx.doi.org/10.1016/B978-0-12-811189-5.00004-0

This chapter offers you the opportunity *to assess what type of culture your organization has today.* It is critical to know what culture you have so that you can identify what changes need to be made.

We realize that you may not be able to do all of it. Everyone, however, can impact culture change. This chapter also offers a *proactive look at how you, in your role, can impact cultural change.*

Our goal is to provide you with an understanding of the desired objectives and how to make a difference in your organization's pursuit of Food Safety. In order to apply the outlined *Roadmap* to culture change within your organization, we will describe things *you can do,* based on the scope of your role, within your organization. We will describe what you can do within your position to impact cultural readiness to fully embrace the principles and tenets of a solid Food Safety initiative. It will help you understand how to do your part to integrate Food Safety fully into your strategy.

Remember to be patient if the situation allows. Convincing people to change sometimes takes time. You may need to plant seeds and give them enough attention and time to actually take root and grow. You should do everything possible to take the necessary time to get it right. However, if you believe you are facing a critical situation, you won't have time to be patient, and your tactics will be much more urgent.

WHAT TYPE OF CULTURE EXISTS IN YOUR ORGANIZATION?

Let's look at the three cultures within an organization, *leading, trending,* and *mentioning.* They span from highly developed to less developed. Read each one and ask yourself, honestly, where do you see your culture? Carefully consider each element listed in the description to see if it pertains to you. You may be some combination of these. If that is the case, you will want to use the least developed one when looking at other matrices about how to deal with culture.

WHICH BEST DESCRIBES YOUR CULTURE?

- *Leading—It Totally Matters Around Here...*

Your organization emphasizes Food Safety throughout the organization. The elements of Food Safety are fully integrated in all departments, at all levels and within all work. Decisions are made with Food Safety in mind. Leaders consistently hold their teams accountable for the correct actions. Measurements are in place. Compliance is recognized, regularly and often. Noncompliance is thoroughly addressed. People do the right thing, even when they are not being watched. They are engaged in the culture and own the outcomes. They avoid just "checking off the boxes." Operators understand the value of a strong emphasis on Food Safety.

- *Trending—We Talk About It a Lot...*

Your organization talks about Food Safety often. The elements of Food Safety are somewhat understood by some members of your organization. Decisions, however, are made more with profit in mind. Leaders do not consistently hold their teams accountable for the correct actions. Some measurements are in place. Compliance is sometimes recognized. Noncompliance is not consistently addressed. People talk about it more than they actually do it. There is awareness and discussion, but not enough ownership.

To move out of this culture into one that is leading, place an emphasis on proactively managing risk. Benchmark to find programs that work and define the gap you have between where you are currently, and where you strive to be. You will know you are making progress when behavior changes from talk to action. You may wish to get third-party assistance with setting up a plan to bridge the gap.

- *Mentioning—We Have Other Concerns...*

A few people in your organization mention Food Safety. The elements of Food Safety handling are not very well understood by most members of your organization. You often hear "We've never had a problem before..."; "It's too expensive"; It's not worth the money"; "We'll take the chance"; or "That's overkill." Decisions do not take Food Safety into consideration. Leaders do not hold their teams accountable for the correct actions. Measurements are not in place. Compliance is rarely recognized and may be disincented. Noncompliance is not addressed. People care more about productivity and profit than anything related to Food Safety.

To move toward a more trending culture, talk about it with everyone. This will enable your organization to be closer to determining what to do and how to do it.

You may find you have a hybrid situation. Perhaps you are trying, and people are talking about Food Safety, but there are still some concerns in the actions of work teams throughout the organization. Maybe you have done all the right things to implement change but nobody is following.

If these situations exist in your organization, pay close attention to how all things in the *Roadmap* are progressing. Keep a constant gage on your actions and frequently adjust your plan and direction when needed. Food Safety should be an agenda item in leadership, department, and employee meetings. Talk openly about what you are trying to accomplish. Talk about successes. Support people with skills to overcome failures. Be open to ideas. Most importantly, be flexible in the way you look at your plan.

WHICH LEVEL ARE YOU?

First you will need to define your role/level within the organization, using the chart below.

This model outlines several options to define your role. Pick the one that most closely resembles where your position falls within the corporate structure. In some cases, you may refer to more than one role for ideas on how to move forward.

Level	Description
C-level	You are the CEO or you report directly to the CEO on his/her Executive Leadership Team. Positions might include: • COO (Operations) • CMO (Marketing and Sales) • CFO (Finance) • CPO (People) • CIO (IT) *C-level leaders who directly manage Directors may want to look at this section, as well as the one titled VP.*
Vice President (VP)	• You have the title of VP and/or you have the responsibility of being closely involved in strategic direction for the company and full authority for the area you oversee • You lead a large segment of the business and are responsible for its results • You primarily manage leaders of leaders (Directors who manage Managers) • You report to a C-level leader, other than the CEO, such as a COO *VPs, who report to the CEO, directly may want to look at this section, as well as the one titled C-level.*
Director	• You have the title of Director and/or you have the responsibility for making sure that the actions of your team support the goals of the company • You oversee a department within the business and are responsible for its results • You primarily manage leaders of employees or Project Managers • You report to a VP *Directors who directly manage individual contributors or workers may want to look at this section, as well as the one titled Manager.*
Manager	• You have the title of Manager, Supervisor or Lead • You manage the work of a team, around goals set for you by your boss and are directly responsible for the work completed by your team • You primarily manage independent contributors or hourly employees • You report to another Director or another Manager *Managers of Managers may want to look at this section, as well as the one titled Director.*

Level	Description
Independent contributor/ employee	• Titles at this level vary • Your job includes work that is a part of a process or project • You do not manage anyone. You are responsible for your own work, but may work within a team responsible for specific goals • You report to a Manager, Supervisor or Team Lead *You may be a Project Manager, in which case, you may want to look at this section, as well as the one titled Manager.*

WHAT AM I TRYING TO DO?

The Figure below outlines the six steps to intentionally shift culture, a graphic representation of the roadmap from Chapter 3.

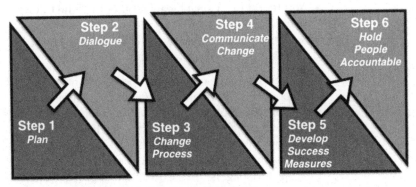

Six-step Roadmap to Intentionally Shift Culture.

Remember the things that need to be done to ensure that culture changes in your organization to support Food Safety. They are the six steps in the process to change culture to more fully embrace Food Safety. They make up the *Roadmap* for culture change and they include the following.

1. *Plan: Integrate Food Safety into your strategic initiatives/ goals.* If Food Safety is not included in your overall Strategic/ Business Goals, it will not materialize or be seen as important in the organization, creating a dangerous situation. Integration provides the foundation necessary to prompt change in your culture to support your goals.

   a. For the purposes of this chapter, your goal is to influence the realization by others that planning is needed and that the plan should visibly include Food Safety.

2. *Dialogue: Get People talking about Food Safety; make it top of mind.* This usually follows the integration of Food Safety into your organization's strategy. It can also be the reason people start to think about doing more about Food Safety. If nothing is happening, get people talking. If things are starting to happen, get them talking more.

   a. *Your goal is to start conversations.* Talk about things that affect Food Safety. Tell stories to which people can relate. Give examples of recalls; share articles from newspapers or magazines on Food Safety. Get them interested. Ask questions. Add Food Safety to agendas. Have an elevator speech in place, a 2–3-sentence description of Food Safety and why it is important to the company. Share your thoughts with everyone you can.

3. *Change Process: Figure out what needs to change to bridge the gap between where you are and what you are trying to accomplish.* If you are a technical person, this will be right up your alley. Plan what needs to change. If you are not a technical person, be sure to include the technical Food Safety experts in your discussion.

   a. *Your goal is to facilitate process change.* This means you will be making sure process change happens effectively, across all parts of the organization that must make changes for improvement. Make people feel they have the power to shut down a line if they see a Food Safety issue. Empower ownership at all levels and in all departments.

4. *Communicate Change: Make sure everyone knows what to do, why they are doing it, and how to complete it the correct way.* Remember, process change does not just include planning to figure out what to do. Successful change is based on effectively communicating the changes.
   a. *Your goal is to build a teaching organization in order to support the changes.* Help people understand how to communicate the importance of change to others. Be sure there is effective education about the reason for the changes. Finally, make sure everyone who must actually change, fully understands how to do so.

Teaching = Education + Training

5. *Develop Success Measures: Set the stage for the game to be played correctly.* Make sure there is an effective means of measuring what affects the desired outcomes of the changes. Be sure you can determine whether the desired actions are actually taking place. Measures will shape culture. Another way to look at this is to ask yourself how you would spot the characteristics offered in Chapter 4—"What Is an Effective Food Safety Culture?"
   a. *Your goal is to influence the willingness to measure the right things.* You may need assistance from people who regularly work with metrics. You will likely find that some metrics are available already, but you may need to develop some to get the most solid indicators.
6. *Implement and Hold Accountable: Begin the culture change when you change and monitor process.* Measures will point to the effectiveness of the change. Leaders should:
   a. Reward positive movement
   b. Hold employees accountable if the desired change is not taking place.
      i. *Your goal is to influence willingness to hold people accountable for the desired changes.*

The following tables make some recommendations for you, based on the type of culture you have and the role you hold. The assumption here is that you believe this is the right thing to do. The table will provide you with specific actions you can take, based on your role, in each of the six major steps below.

Remember the steps are:

- *Plan*
- *Dialog*
- *Change Process*
- *Communicate Change*
- *Develop Success Measures*
- *Implement and Hold Accountable.*

To use the table, first find the one for your level. Next find the type of culture you think you have. Review the recommended actions listed. If you find that you are in one culture for some of the steps, but haven't started the others, start in the furthest left box to see the progression you can take to reach the ultimate end goal. The suggestions under the "Mentioning Culture" help you get started. The suggestions under "Trending Culture" help you gain momentum. The suggestions under "Leading Culture" help you achieve a higher level of excellence.

Finally, share this book with everyone involved.

C-Level

You can very likely make the decisions. You can make this happen. You can change things very quickly. You will gain great benefits by moving forward. You also have the most to lose if you don't.

Roadmap	Mentioning Culture	Trending Culture	Leading Culture
Steps	You have a way to go, but it's possible! Start here.	You have started, but you aren't quite there, yet.	Keep Doing What Your'e Doing And…
1. Plan Goal: influence to get planning to happen	Learn everything you can about planning and provide opportunities for your team to do the same. Challenge teams to develop a strong plan to include the integration of Food Safety into your day-to-day approach to business. Outside facilitation is highly recommended. Once you address Food Safety, you can expand your planning to become more strategic on other areas.	Require planning to take place for the organization, as a whole and then within each department. Require plans to be very specific about how Food Safety will be addressed differently. Outside facilitation is very helpful to get this started. You may also wish to consider training on the methods and means of planning.	You likely have a plan. Be sure that planning continues to take place and is focused on integrating Food Safety. Likely, planning will address other strategic initiatives, as well. Keep planning on all areas top of mind, regular and evolving. Outside facilitation can push your leaders to plan for a higher level of excellence than you currently experience.
2. Dialogue Goal: start conversations	Start by asking questions at meetings. Show people you want to make a change in how work is done. Ask them to consider what they think needs to change. Challenge them to consider what could happen if the organization does not get more serious about this.	Include Food Safety on every agenda as a standing item to review progress, shortcomings, and solutions to barriers. Regularly talk about what is needed. Talk openly about risk and the mitigation the organization can do.	Ask your leaders to give you input on how to raise the bar to an even higher level. Ask specific questions to make sure this is on meeting agendas, regularly.

3. Change Process Goal: facilitate process change	If you have a person in charge of Food Safety that is technically competent, ask them to provide you with a list of recommendations. If you do not, seek input from a qualified outside provider.	Consult regularly with your Food Safety staff to review process challenges and leverage their recommendations across other departments. A qualified outside provider can assist you in making sure you have thought of everything.	You likely follow good process. Be sure problems are being identified and handled effectively and quickly.
4. Communicate Change Goal: build a teaching organization	Training will likely be needed. Identify all resources who can assist in communicating. Walk your team through the details of an effective change communication plan. Let them shape the plan. Challenge them to fully implement the plan.	Once needed changes are clearly identified, be sure your leaders develop a formal change communication plan. Be sure they follow it. Training may be needed to ensure the best communication and teaching.	Most organizations don't do this well without some intentional focus. Hold others accountable for making change communication a priority. Ask your leaders for comprehensive Communication Plans. Make sure they are detailed enough to support change. Training may be needed to ensure the best communication and teaching.
5. Develop Success Measures Goal: influence willingness to measure	Analyze currently measured items to see what they actually tell you about your organization. Ask enough questions to see what is missing. If your organization has not used a lot of metrics, some training may be needed.	Identify the right measures to tell you if change is actually occurring. Remember that culture is what's measured around here—so shifting from no measures or the wrong measures to the right measures will pave the way for change to stick. Set up tracking and monitor measures regularly.	You likely already have measures. Be sure you are measuring the right things. Be sure measures are being watched and monitored and that they actually measure success.

Roadmap	Mentioning Culture	Trending Culture	Leading Culture
6. Implement and Hold Accountable Goal: influence willingness to ensure change happens	Start with training your leaders and managers to hold people accountable and to recognize performance. If you already do this well, be sure they understand how to articulate expectations to each person on their team. This will be the vehicle by which you can achieve implementation. The process of holding a person accountable prompts culture change.	Set up tracking to monitor compliance to the new process. Learn to use the measures as a prompt to recognize a person through some form of reward, when applicable. Also, learn to use the measures to correct actions and hold others accountable. Some training to do this with others may be needed for your leaders and their managers to hold others accountable.	Inspect what you expect, as the saying goes. Spot check. Ask questions. Look at the possibility of adding Leadership Development Programs or Management Training to help leaders with their skills in holding others accountable. Make sure your rewards programs are on target with your goals.
Remember	As a C-level leader, you can immediately impact change. Your words and actions are likely watched and followed. When you talk about this at your level, it impresses upon others that this is a priority, simply because you hold a top-level position. Don't just talk; your actions will speak louder. Integrate Food Safety fully into your Strategic Plan. Make it a priority and call people to action, regularly.		

Vice President Level

You can heavily influence your teams to embrace this. Your position can gain total commitment from your team, so your challenge will be to influence others at your level to do the same. You can also influence upward to get the C-level leaders to get more involved. Some of the recommendations mirror that of the C-level. You can directly impact your teams, but may need to work harder to impact other teams headed by other VPs.

Roadmap	Mentioning Culture	Trending Culture	Leading Culture
Steps	You have a way to go, but it's possible! Start here.	You have started, but you aren't quite there, yet.	Keep Doing What Your'e Doing And…
1. Plan Goal: influence to get planning to happen	Influence C-level leaders that planning should take place. Be sure that you bring up this issue as a consideration. Outside facilitation is highly recommended. Once you address Food Safety, you can expand your planning to become more strategic in other areas.	Be sure plans are very specific about how Food Safety will be addressed differently. Outside facilitation is very helpful to get this started. You may also wish to consider training on the methods and means of planning.	Contribute to your organization's strategy. Challenge the people who work for you to develop comprehensive action plans to accomplish strategy within their departments.
2. Dialogue Goal: start conversations	Ask questions. Start talking. Start by asking questions at meetings. Show people you want to make a change in how work is done. Ask them to consider what they think needs to change. Challenge them to consider what could happen if the organization does not get more serious about this.	Include Food Safety on the agenda for every meeting you hold, as a formal agenda item to review progress, shortcomings and solutions to barriers. Regularly talk about what is needed. Talk openly about risk and the mitigation that the organization can do.	Make sure Food Safety is talked about at all of your meetings and ask your people to do the same. Ask people specific questions during walk-throughs and in one-on-one meetings.

3. Change Process Goal: facilitate process change	If you run an area that directly manages process related to Food Safety, ask your teams to evaluate their process. Involve your technical experts in Food Safety and ask them to provide you with a list of recommendations. If you do not have such a person in your organization, seek this input from a qualified outside provider. If you do not run an area responsible for Food Safety process but feel your organization needs to take a deeper look, utilize your influence skills to address the situation.	Consult regularly with your Food Safety staff to review process challenges and leverage their recommendations across other departments. A qualified outside provider can assist you in making sure you have thought of everything.	Be active in making sure that process is continually reviewed for efficiency and effectiveness. Be sure problems are being identified and handled effectively and quickly.
4. Communicate Change Goal: build a teaching organization	Training will likely be needed. Identify all resources who can assist in communicating. Walk your team through the details of an effective change communication plan. Let them shape the plan. Challenge them to implement the plan, fully. Establish common language about what should be communicated, and the definition of teaching.	Once the needed changes are clearly identified, be sure your leaders develop a formal change communication plan. Be sure they follow it. Training may be needed to ensure the best communication and teaching. You will also want to influence your peers to do the same.	Challenge your organization to measure and be sure the measures are accurate, timely and communicated well. Monitor them regularly. Talk about them and help others understand how to use them.

Roadmap	Mentioning Culture	Trending Culture	Leading Culture
5. Develop Success Measures Goal: influence willingness to measure	Analyze currently measured items to see what they actually tell you about your organization. Ask enough questions to begin to see what is missing. If your organization has not used a lot of metrics, some training may be needed.	Identify the right measures to tell you if change is actually occurring. Remember that culture is what's measured around here—so shifting from no measures or the wrong measures to the right measures will pave the way for change to stick. Set up tracking and monitor measures regularly.	Communicate all aspects of the change to people offering education, training, and skills development as needed. Be sure goals are not mutually exclusive.
6. Implement and Hold Accountable Goal: influence willingness to ensure change happens	Start with training your leaders and managers to hold people accountable and to recognize performance. If you already do this well, be sure they understand how to articulate expectations to each person on their team. This will be the vehicle by which you can achieve implementation. The process of holding a person accountable prompts culture change.	Set up tracking to monitor compliance to the new process. Learn to use the measures as a prompt to recognize a person through some form of reward, when applicable. Also, learn to use the measures to correct actions and hold others accountable. Some training to do this with others may be needed for your leaders and their managers to hold others accountable.	Hold people accountable for change. Be sure people are doing the work, even when their bosses aren't looking. Highlight any problems you see for immediate resolution.
Remember	As a VP, you will need to influence organizational strategy but ensure departmental execution. You and your peers, together, can develop the answers. Work with them. Involve them. Be sure to gain commitment from your C-level if needed in order to get the support you are looking for.		

Director Level

You can challenge your people to embrace change. You can influence others to embrace it, also. Most of your success will rest with your ability to present a strong case in the language of the person who can actually make a change. Don't be hesitant to ask your VP for training, where you need to develop your skills.

Roadmap Steps	Mentioning Culture	Trending Culture	Leading Culture
1. Plan Goal: influence to get planning to happen	You have a way to go, but it's possible! Start here.	You have started, but you aren't quite there, yet.	Keep Doing What Your'e Doing And…
	Present a strong case to build the realization that not doing a plan puts the organization at a very high risk. Prepare your case for planning. Talk the language of the person you are presenting to. Include measures and metrics.	Ask people if they have a plan for Food Safety. Develop your own plan. Develop a plan to change what you can. Take advantage of autonomy you might have. Spread enthusiasm about what you think needs to be done.	Be strategic in the way you run your department. Be sure the day-to-day activity is tied into what your organization is trying to accomplish.
2. Dialogue Goal: start conversations	Build a strong case for a stronger Food Safety culture. Start dropping pieces of this case in conversations wherever possible. Start a buzz; create a movement of discovery.	Ask questions. Talk openly. Challenge thinking. Add Food Safety to your agendas. Get people to discover needs through your questions.	Make sure Food Safety is talked about at all of your meetings and ask your people to do the same. Ask people specific questions during walk-throughs and in 1:1 meetings.
3. Change Process Goal: facilitate process change	Identify the process change you can directly impact or influence. Encourage your peers to do the same.	Change the process you can impact. Encourage your peers to do the same.	Challenge process. Highlight any problems you see for immediate resolution.

4. Communicate Change Goal: build a teaching organization	Begin to influence others as to the need for change communication. Highlight examples of times when not doing good change management hindered positive flow of work in the organization.	Seek out learning and development to be a strong teacher. Teach your managers to do the same. Be sure to communicate any changes you plan, proactively and before they occur. Follow up with education to help them understand why something should be done and training to help them understand how the work will be different.	Communicate, educate, train and develop skills wherever possible. Always be teaching. Make sure your managers are developing a system to track their communication to be sure everyone gets the necessary information.
5. Develop Success Measures Goal: influence willingness to measure	Determine how you will be able to tell if you and your team are accomplishing the changes you are making.	Ask what measures are available to you, prompting better measures that can really help you assess whether or not the process changes you are targeting are happening.	Review measures regularly and take action to reward or correct in a timely fashion.
6. Implement and Hold Accountable Goal: influence willingness to ensure change happens	Hold people accountable for change. Help them improve.	Hold people accountable for change. Help them improve.	Hold people accountable for change. Help them improve.
Remember	As a Director, you are responsible for connecting the work of your people to the goals of the future. You can influence upward and outward to your peers. You have more direct control over the teams you direct.		

Manager Level

You manage the people that need to make the changes. Be sure they are doing things that are needed. You will notice that some of your recommendations mirror those of a Director, because you can do them for the areas you oversee. Don't be hesitant to ask your boss for training where you think it will benefit you.

Roadmap	Mentioning Culture	Trending Culture	Leading Culture
Steps	You have a way to go, but it's possible! Start here.	You have started, but you aren't quite there, yet.	Keep Doing What Your'e Doing And…
1. Plan Goal: influence to get planning to happen	Present a strong case to build the realization that not doing a plan puts the organization at a very high risk. Prepare your case for planning. Talk the language of the person you are presenting to. Include measures and metrics.	Ask people if they have a plan for Food Safety. Develop your own plan. Develop a plan to change what you can. Take advantage of autonomy you might have. Spread enthusiasm about what you think needs to be done.	Be strategic in the way you run your department. Be sure the day-to-day activity is tied into what your organization is trying to accomplish.
2. Dialogue Goal: start conversations	Build a strong case for a stronger culture in Food Safety. Start dropping pieces of this case in conversations wherever possible. Start a buzz; create a movement of discovery.	Ask questions. Talk openly. Challenge thinking. Add Food Safety to your agendas. Get people to discover needs through your questions.	Make sure Food Safety is talked about at all of your meetings and ask your people to do the same. Ask people specific questions during walk-throughs and in 1:1 meetings.
3. Change Process Goal: facilitate process change	Identify the process change you can directly impact or influence. Encourage your peers to do the same.	Change the process you can impact. Encourage your peers to do the same.	Challenge process. Highlight any problems you see for immediate resolution.

4. Communicate Change Goal: build a teaching organization	Begin to influence others as to the need for change communication. Highlight examples of times when not doing good change management hindered positive flow of work in the organization.	Seek out learning and development to be a strong teacher. Teach your managers to do the same. Be sure to communicate any changes you plan, proactively and before they occur. Follow up with education to help them understand why something should be done and training to help them understand how the work will be different.	Communicate, educate, train, and develop skills wherever possible. This job will rest heavily on you. Be sure you develop systems to track to be sure everyone receives what they need.
5. Develop Success Measures Goal: influence willingness to measure	Determine how you will be able to tell if you and your team are accomplishing the changes you are making.	Ask what measures are available to you, prompting better measures that can really help you assess whether or not the process changes you are targeting are happening.	Review measures regularly and take action to reward or correct in a timely fashion.
6. Implement and Hold Accountable Goal: influence willingness to ensure change happens	Hold people accountable for change. Help them improve.	Hold people accountable for change. Help them improve.	Hold people accountable for change. Help them improve.
Remember	As a Manager, you are ensuring the work is being done correctly.		

Individual Contributor

You are where the rubber meets the road. If you don't make changes, they won't happen. Your goals are likely to be different from the Managers, Directors, or VPs. You need to understand what you need to do, but you also need to point out to others what might need to be done.

This table deals with the individual contributor outside of Food Safety. If you oversee Food Safety, and you do not have a team you manage, still follow the guidelines listed in the Director and Manager tables. Your role likely influences the rest of the organization from that level, even though you don't have direct reports.

Roadmap Steps	Mentioning Culture	Trending Culture	Leading Culture
	You have a way to go, but it's possible! Start here.	You have started, but you aren't quite there, yet.	Keep Doing What Your'e Doing And...
1. Plan Goal: understand	Ask if there is a plan.	Provide input to help get a plan moving through your Manager.	Ask to see the plan if you haven't already. Offer suggestions to share the elements of the plan with your peers.
2. Dialogue Goal: start conversations	Ask questions about things that concern you.	Make suggestions about things that concern you.	Contribute your ideas at staff meetings where Food Safety is being talked about.
3. Change Process Goal: recommend improvement	Make suggestions about processes you think could or should change.	Make specific recommendations about ways that change could better support Food Safety.	Process has likely been changed. Share input where you have it. Highlight any problems you see with ideas for solutions.
4. Communicate Change Goal: adapt to the change	Make sure you know what to do. Ask questions when you don't know what to do.	Make sure you know what to do. Ask questions when you don't know what to do.	Make sure you know what to do. Ask questions when you don't know what to do.

5. Develop Success Measures Goal: understand measures	Ask how you know if you are doing a good job.	Ask how your performance will be measured.	Look at the metrics available to you regularly. Understand what they are telling you.
6. Implement and Hold Accountable Goal: do your part; challenge your peers	Follow process and hold peers accountable to do the same.	Follow process and hold peers accountable to do the same.	Follow process and hold peers accountable to do the same.
Remember	You are doing the work. Take pride in it. Point out things that make it difficult to you. Point out anything you have concerns about.		

As we move to the next section, we will explore gaining commitment and momentum at all levels. You can't change culture without influencing commitment. You can't influence commitment without changing culture.

Another way to look at culture is to understand that it is a combination of your best science, with solid management and supported by effective communication.

Culture = Best Science + Solid Management + Effective Communication

This section introduced a six-step process for culture change that comprises the *Roadmap* for culture change. In order to achieve it, you will need commitment. If you can't demand it, you will need to influence it. In the next section, we will offer specific tips to speak the language of the person you need to influence in order to successfully present your case and gain their full commitment.

Section II

Gaining Solid Organizational Commitment

Chapter 5

How to Influence Commitment

Chapter Outline

WHAT IS COMMITMENT?

According to Webster, commitment is defined as *"the state or quality of being dedicated to a cause."* Synonyms include words like *guarantee, promise, pledge,* and *responsibility.* The implication is that once committed, a person has decided to put forth all resources to do what he or she must to ensure the desired outcome.

To fully integrate the strategic initiative of Food Safety into an organization, full commitment is required. All employees, at every level, should be dedicated to doing everything within their power to ensure that food is grown, processed, prepared, handled, merchandized, and distributed properly so that the customer and consumer have the lowest possible risk of illness.

Interestingly, Webster's second definition of commitment is "an engagement or obligation that restricts freedom of action." Once committed, people may have to change their behaviors and, in doing so, they lose the freedom to do things the way they used to do them. To fully integrate Food Safety into an organization, employees are no longer free to do what they want, such as take shortcuts or disregard the important aspects of Food Safety.

Food Safety. DOI: http://dx.doi.org/10.1016/B978-0-12-811189-5.00005-2

Commitment and culture are endlessly interconnected. Yet, they are different things.

Commitment is a decision or choice. Every person in the organization must support the integration of Food Safety into the organization.

Culture is an environment. It demands adherence to the right actions, regardless of whether or not anyone is looking.

Commitment is measured by actions. Positive, appropriate actions indicate commitment. Negative actions and failure to uphold standards indicate a lack of commitment.

Culture exists because actions are measured. Positive, appropriate actions are recognized and rewarded, showing everyone that *"This is the way we do things around here."* Negative actions and failure to uphold standards are addressed with consequences and accountability, showing everyone that *"Not doing the right things is simply not acceptable."*

Commitment is a critical ingredient to create culture. It is the belief on the part of each individual in your organization that it is important.

Culture cannot sustain itself without *commitment*.

Commitment cannot sustain itself in the absence of a supporting *culture*.

Commitment is influenced. It is a choice on the part of each individual in the organization to believe in the "cause" and to do the "right thing."

Culture is defined. It sets the expectations.

Both commitment and culture involve communication to the members of your organization as well as the measurement of their actions. We have previously referred to communication, measurement, and accountability as the "glue" in the puzzle.

HOW TO GET COMMITMENT...

Remember that true commitment is needed from everyone: senior leadership; all managers and supervisors; and all employees who do the work. Getting commitment sounds simple, but it requires influence. The top person in an organization or department should just be able to say "Food Safety is important," and everyone will jump on board. Right?

We all know it doesn't happen that way, much to the dismay and frustration of many top leaders. Instead, commitment will require influence. People will need to be convinced to change their behavior and maybe even persuaded to change the way they think. Minds will need to be shifted in order to fully shift commitment from "paying lip service" to Food Safety to actually being driven to make it the best it can possibly be.

Keeping commitment requires leaders to hold their people accountable for making the necessary changes. They will need to reward good performance and correct (firmly) when people don't do the right things. A "glue" ingredient, once again, so commitment will occur and change will happen.

Leaders must believe in and consistently communicate change in ways that inspire others. This is a leadership skill that takes work. Leaders who make it a priority to learn how to do this get better over time.

The ability to get commitment requires you to influence
people, every day.
This must occur in order to shape culture.
This must be present to impact change.

So, if influence is the best way to get commitment, regardless of the level of position you hold, everyone reading this book and everyone you share it with can participate. The best way to gain commitment is to effectively use influence to persuade people to believe in doing the right thing, and develop a strong enough commitment so they won't do the wrong thing or overlook something that is contrary to good Food Safety. If the organization has utilized a strong communication plan in conjunction with the effort, it sets the stage to make your job of influencing someone easier. In order to really influence change, you must understand what is important to the other person and recognize how their language may be different from your own.

Before we discuss the elements within the skill of influencing others better, let's take a look at the merits of being able to do it. Not only will it support this effort, but also just about everything you do in your job and your personal life requires you to be good at influencing others. Influence can help you convince others to change or try something different. It can get others to buy into your ideas. Influence is a critical skill necessary to sell anything. Influence is necessary for effective leadership. The ability to influence others is a skill that most of us aren't born with, but develop throughout our lifetime.

FIRST, UNDERSTAND BUSINESS PRIORITIES

When utilizing communication and influence to impact the viewpoint of someone else in a different department or at a different level, always keep in mind the goals for which they are accountable. Position your influence point to be able to support their goals. For example, if you are trying to influence someone in Operations who is accountable for a particular number (eg, amount of product produced in a specific timeframe), present your case in a way that helps them see how their numbers are important and how what you are requiring will positively impact this measure.

Let's take a deeper look at the business priorities by department and the impact Food Safety can have on that department's goals. This information is necessary to effectively influence change. If you don't have a clear understanding of the business and what drives decisions, you will not be able to influence them.

Department	What Do They Care About?	How Can Food Safety Help Them?
Operations	<ul><li>Fulfillment accuracy</li><li>Fulfillment cycle time</li><li>Productivity</li><li>Return on working capital</li><li>Cycle time to ship</li></ul>	<ul><li>Fewer rejections</li><li>Better yield</li><li>Reduced cycle time</li><li>Less problems</li><li>Ability to meet new product requests in a timely and effective manner</li></ul>
Purchasing	<ul><li>Cost</li><li>Yield</li><li>Quality of materials</li></ul>	<ul><li>Consistency</li><li>Better yield</li><li>Fewer rejections</li><li>Just-in-time planning</li><li>Ensures quality suppliers</li></ul>

Department	What Do They Care About?	How Can Food Safety Help Them?
Sales	• Revenue • Customer satisfaction	• Fewer complaints • Less returns • Consistently meet orders • Improved satisfaction
Marketing	• Brand awareness • Flexibility to meet market place needs	• Improved brand perception • Speed of marketing execution • Minimized risk; greater confidence across company and consumers
R&D	• Goals for new product development	• Minimized risk; quicker to market • Ensures quality suppliers
Distribution	• Quality of shipment • Accuracy of shipment	• Less returns
HR	• Retention • Recruiting • Training	• Improved retention due to better job satisfaction • Enhanced recruiting due to quality commitment • Improved education and training to support Food Safety, which transfers over to other strategic initiatives • Better change management
Finance	• Bottom line	• Proven positive impact on bottom line • Reduced chance for expenses in recalls
C-Level	• Profit and loss (P&L) • Strategic plan	• Assists in meeting P&L • Reduced risk of recall having an impact on stock price, brand equity, morale, and legal obligations
All departments	• Goals	• Less recalls • Customer/consumer safety • Pride

Remember that Food Safety is an insurance policy that drives value. Don't immediately think that you must speak about return on investment (ROI). Rather, emphasize that it is the right thing to do and demonstrate your knowledge of what it will cost to do it effectively. Think about how what you are asking for affects the total bottom line. Compel yourself to look beyond the obvious. Learn and know enough about other departments and systems to effectively communicate in terms they will understand. For example, understand the financial reports on which decisions are made in sufficient detail to be able to relate to the impact of effective Food Safety programs on those numbers. This can be enhanced if you have a financial person as part of the Food Safety Team or Steering Committee.

To further reiterate the need to make a business case for the change you believe to be necessary, let's explore the concept of Predictive Financial Thinking (PFT). PFT is what influences departmental leaders to make decisions. The term itself focuses on connecting the science to the business case with a logical framework that the business leader can fully understand. Demonstrate that you are willing to understand the impact on the business (both cost and efficiency) and that you are willing to do the work to demonstrate a Return on Investment (ROI).

Remember to demonstrate competency in your communications with the departments that will need to support change in order to improve your organization's commitment to Food Safety. Be sure to remain objective. Don't expect them to do the right thing simply because it is the right thing. You have to show them why.

NEXT, UNDERSTAND THE TWO DIFFERENT PERSPECTIVES OF RISK

The next difference to understand is the differing perspectives about risk, between technical professionals in Food Safety and the primary perspective held by many decision makers in the organization. Remember, Risk = Severity + Probability. Food Safety technical professionals usually think about risk in terms of severity, while the rest of the organization's leadership is more likely to think about risk in terms of probability. Since risk is really defined as severity plus probability, both are partially right. This simple difference in perspective about risk can often lead to difficulties/disconnects in a team's ability to develop solutions that will positively impact Food Safety. Additionally, the technical people may have difficulty in building credibility when communicating with the non-technical people, due to this difference. This can also impact the credibility of the technical people as exemplified with often-heard complaints such as "Technical people always think the sky is falling"; or "They don't understand the business".

Think about what is implied within this difference. In Food Safety, the technical professional is working to mitigate severity. This requires a focus on the possible different scenarios in which severity can increase, most of which are based on speculation about worst-case scenarios. This is their job. Likely, this creates a level of emotional concern in the mind of the Food Safety professional that may not be matched by his/her nontechnical counterpart. To them, it is so clear that these potential problems are worth mitigating, but the non-technical management team may not see it that way. They are more interested in probability. They may have less sense of urgency about the potential scenarios, or the probability that something could go wrong, particularly if nothing major has gone wrong, yet.

When these two perspectives about risk clash, the Food Safety professional often does not understand why leadership is not seeing the problems inherent in the potential severity and may think they don't care. Additionally, technical professionals see things in very clear, concrete terms (black and white) and may not be willing to or understand how to explore the gray areas of "No" to get to a solution that can work. The leadership team may think that the Food Safety message is based on too much speculation and overstated, or that they are not willing to work through different solutions to find the right solution. These differences can be overcome if both parties engage in enough dialog to review facts that back up the concepts of severity and probability.

Food Safety professionals need to be mindful of how they come across. Since their perspective is rooted in science and is concrete in how they view it, they may be prone to showcasing intellect, or taking a stand of compliance and oversight, when collaboration is a better course of action. Research for this book often pointed to the fact that when a Food Safety professional takes an alarmist point of view, the organization may not take them seriously. Effective communication is the way that you control issues before they occur.

HOW TO INFLUENCE OTHERS BY UNDERSTANDING THEIR LANGUAGE

If your organization is already committed to Food Safety as a critical and imperative strategic initiative, your job is easier. Your influence efforts to gain commitment will be directed toward making sure people commit to meeting the expectations.

If they have not started yet, you will need to start your influence efforts by trying to gain commitment to the importance of changing expectations. Remember, no matter how far along your organization is in building a commitment to culture change, everything you can do to influence the change will help bring it further along.

Even though influence is dealt with as a part of this section on commitment, it is part of the glue necessary to bring all of the parts together. *Influence* is the art of changing the way a person thinks. The goal of influence is to convince people to change their behavior.

There are some key elements to influencing others. The first thing we must do to influence effectively is realize that not everyone processes information in the same way. Thus, influence will require us to package/present our point of view into the other person's language so that they receive it in ways that make sense to them. *We must remember that it is not about us; it is about them.*

There are four steps to influencing others.

The information below is excerpted from "Judge Not, A Guide to Influence People Who Think Differently" by Patti Leith, © by EDGES, Inc.

1. Spot/notice that there is a difference.

     About half of the world considers themselves to be *similar* to others. If you fall into this category, you are likely unassuming and approachable. With little or no arrogance, you go about your business feeling like you identify with the world. This is good on most fronts, but the downside to this characteristic (every characteristic has an upside and a downside) is that you will expect others to react as you would. So much so, you may be very surprised when they don't; so much so, it may take you a while to realize that a difference exists.

Even though you probably conceptually realize everyone is different, and you are okay with that, you are likely to overlook difference when you are faced with it. You won't be able to change this feeling of similarity to others, nor should you try. You should, however, be able to spot key signs a person is not responding to things the way that you would. This is your clue to adjust.

The other half of the world considers themselves to be *unique*. If you fall into this group, you know others are different, and are probably proud of how you are different. The first step is noticing the difference. Since you will be looking for it, it will be easy for you. You will conceptually prepare yourself for people to respond differently than you do, and not be surprised when they do. Your pride in your own approach, however, may cause you to judge them more quickly.

2. Know what that difference is…

Insight into yourself and others is key to this process, as is the ability to check your biases at the door. You must be attuned to behaviors that tell you about the people around you, and be able to accept them for who they are in order for this to work. You must be very aware of the approaches you bring to the table—another key ingredient for the success of this process. Some of us are born with good insight, while others do not naturally read others well. If you do not naturally read others well, look for differences in their behavior as compared to yours. There are three things that significantly impact a person's language or way of communicating about things.

- How do they approach work? What is the level of structure they use when doing work?
  - Ask yourself if they are more structured than you or less structured.
  - Are they more detailed or less detailed in their approach?
- How do they solve problems? What is the level of dialog they have when solving problems?

- o Are they more engaged than you, or are they more intro-
     spective than you?
- o Do they talk when they are figuring something out or are
     they quiet?
- How do they influence others? What is their primary language or approach when influencing others?
  - o Are they more direct than you or more cautious?
  - o Are they honest and up front, or more diplomatic?

3. Now let's look at how to plan a connection to adapt to that
   difference.

   Once you know what is different, it is time to plan how to
   respond to that difference. The guiding rule is that you will try
   to speak their language, unless yours is so strong that you need
   them to help you by understanding yours. There are ways to adapt
   to the things you will be figuring out about that person.

   - How do they approach work? What is the level of structure
     they use when doing work?
     - o If they are more structured than you are, provide more
          detail than you need.
     - o If they are less structured than you are, focus on outcomes
          and results of the effort.
   - How do they solve problems? What is the level of dialog
     they have when solving problems?
     - o If they are more engaged than you, prepare to discuss the
          things they are figuring out.
     - o If they are more introspective than you, give them infor-
          mation you want to talk about in advance.
   - How do they influence others? What is their primary lan-
     guage when influencing others?
     - o If they are more direct than you, keep your points suc-
          cinct and direct.
   - If they are less direct than you, ask questions.

   If you do not think about other people's language differences
   and how to adapt and connect to each other's communication
   styles, your natural or instinctive approach will not reach the
   other person, at least 50% of the time.

4. Keep trying until you see evidence that your message is getting
   through and influencing a change in behavior, or persuading
   the other person to have a change of mind.

DON'T MAKE IT EMOTIONAL... A CASE STUDY

Often, there is some emotion or need that encourages you to influence another person. You care about what you are trying to convince others to do. In the case of Food Safety there is also an ethical component, because if you don't do the right things, innocent people may die or become ill. So, if you are trying to convince someone who believes efforts to do the right thing will impact profit, you may feel like drawing a line in the sand. That, however, almost never works. Once done, the damage may be irreparable.

Consider this situation. A Vice President refuses to make a commitment to a substantial process change that would minimize existing Food Safety risk. The Director under him has been very vocal and attempts three times to convince the Vice President to make the changes. Feeling frustrated, the Director becomes emotional. He refuses to do work the way he believes is incorrect. The vocal Director has a very direct form of communicating. The Vice President and other team members know he is proceeding with change despite the fact that it has not been approved because he believes it will help the company's ability to provide safe food. Everyone also knows that the change will impact the budget and will need approval and support to be sustainable.

The Director refused to continue the process he believed to be wrong. That was a highly ethical commitment, but one that put his presence on the team at risk. He did not further the perceived bad practice. However, he did not influence the Vice President to do the right thing, either. In this situation, the Vice President eventually forced the hand of the Director to switch departments. The Director eventually left the company. The process never changed.

If this person had been less emotional and perhaps more cautious in his influence style, the decision to do what he thought was right without approval may have been less public and certainly would have been more subtle. Such an approach may have even influenced change. When the Director became emotional and espoused his commitment to a "matter of principle," he drew a line in the sand. He set up a battle which he had a high probability of losing.

It could be argued that the Director could never have impacted his Vice President and that the Vice President was too narrow-minded to change. While that may be true, we will argue that the

Director did not try hard enough. When you get emotional and draw a line, your point of view will be known and maybe even applauded by some. Change, however, is not likely to occur. To affect change, you must position your case so you speak the language of the other person you are trying to influence and resonate with his/her job objectives. This takes time, so approach others who can be of assistance, and if necessary, get advice on how to best position your point of view.

Finally, if the change you believe is needed is of critical importance, take your concerns higher in the organization and act immediately. Present the facts, the solutions, and the implications to the company in terms that higher management will understand. In doing so, stay calm, objective, and present a very solid case that highlights the potential impact of doing nothing.

SOME CLOSING THOUGHTS ABOUT INFLUENCE...

The role of the Food Safety professional is to minimize risk for the company. It is not enough to simply know how to do that or to tell others what to do and how to do it. You must convince them that it is needed. You can have the best approach in the world, but it will not be done if you cannot influence or persuade others to buy-in. Influence takes time and energy. For most people, it is a developed skill, rather than an instinct. Your professional development should place the ability to understand how to effectively influence others, front and center. Be a practicing student of influence. Always be learning about it; always be trying new ways to do it. Learn what works for others around you.

Chapter 6

How to Measure Commitment

Chapter Outline

HOW WILL YOU KNOW WHEN YOU HAVE ENOUGH COMMITMENT?

An organization's commitment can always improve. Gaining commitment is a constant effort and a full-time endeavor, requiring focus and attention. The objective for gaining commitment is to have owners, rather than renters. You set expectations, you communicate those expectations and you influence others to follow them. Then, you measure commitment.

Once leadership becomes committed in words and action, they have to pass that down to people in supervisory/management positions. Once those managers and supervisors become committed, they have to pass that down to people on their teams, doing the work. There are often new people coming in. Every day offers another opportunity to build commitment. Every day can also see a loss of commitment or a setback to it. This is most often present in an organization that measures in ways that tempt people to take shortcuts. Gaining commitment is like driving a car. If you fall asleep at the wheel, you will lose control.

Food Safety. DOI: http://dx.doi.org/10.1016/B978-0-12-811189-5.00006-4

THE DESIRED END STATE

The desired end state is achieved when the following occurs:

- Leaders talk openly about problems and solutions.
- There is encouragement to do the right thing.
- There is good compliance to the changed process.
- There is reward and recognition when people do the right thing.
- Noncompliance is addressed with corrective actions, either teaching and/or discipline.
- Food Safety professionals are included in decision-making meetings, with key departments.
  - o Purchasing about equipment design, applicability, etc.
  - o R&D/Product Development about new or modified products/ services.
  - o Marketing about telling others about new or modified products/menu items/services.
  - o Operations about sanitation, pest control, workflow design, workplace design and necessary modifications, etc.
  - o Engineering about plant design or modifications.
- Food Safety professionals should sign off on decisions that have Food Safety implications.
- Situations involving Food Safety are known and understood.
- Food Safety is mentioned in the organization's Mission, Vision, and Strategic Goals.
- Resources (people, money, etc.) for Food Safety are allocated with appropriate justification.
- Departmental cooperation with Food Safety is encouraged and recognized as having a positive impact on the bottom line and in assessment metrics.
- Tasks completed by employees are aligned to the standards set forth by Food Safety.

WAYS TO MEASURE

Measures include more obvious numeric (hard) results such as impact on the business, no recalls, better quality, higher productivity, better cycle time, increased customer/consumer satisfaction, longer shelf life, and better audit scores. Additionally, an increase in commitment to Food Safety should increase pride across the organization, lowering employee turnover and improving morale, both of which are also measurable in numbers.

Less obvious (soft) measures include perceived minimized risk, greater employee involvement and input, better inter- and intradepartmental cooperation, higher respect for management and better problem solving at lower levels in the organization. These are the things that you cannot put a firm number on, but you can see them improve and people will qualitatively reference their improvement.

If you find you are missing some of the "Desired End State" attributes, identify what you need to do to improve it and determine how you can tell when it has improved. These should also be your metrics. Performance Reviews should be a tool to measure that actions are supporting the standards. All required change should be reflected in Job Descriptions and in Process Documentation. This makes expectations clear and also reduces the number of "work-arounds." Work-arounds are problematic because they are simply a band-aid to deal with a less-than-desirable situation which is allowed to remain in place because it has been worked around. This practice in an organization can foster mediocrity and create extremely fragmented processes, which reduce consistency of standards.

RENTERS TO OWNERS

While the organization may not arrive at full commitment, people can. The objective for influencing commitment is to build every member of the organization into an owner's mentality, rather than thinking about their job as a rental. You must work to keep them thinking that way and doing the right thing, even if no one is looking.

Think about the difference between renting and owning. If a pipe backs up, the owner buys plumbing supplies to fix it on their own. They talk to everyone in the house about ways to avoid a reoccurrence and they call in a plumber if they can't fix it themselves. They try and solve the problem, themselves.

Renters, on the other hand, call the landlord to fix the pipes. If the landlord doesn't come, or if he/she doesn't send a plumber, the renter may call again if the situation is inconvenient enough. If it is not causing a problem for them, the renter may let it go, knowing that the consequence of a backed up sink that overflows could cause damage, but that is the landlord's problem, not theirs. The rationale is "I called them and they didn't come out..." There is the dreaded "they" again. Not we; they. The belief that "they will fix it" or "they should be responsible" saps productivity and seriously derails effective responses. They pass the problem off to others to solve.

Who do you want working on your team? Renters who think everyone else should solve their problem? Or, would you rather have owners who take the initiative and do the right things to better the situation, together, immediately?

Culture should support the owner mentality, because it can inspire pride and motivation to do the right thing. Culture can be a very strong component of building the concept of "we." What "we are trying to do" what "we are a part of." Commitment can ensure this, because it influences people about the importance of Food Safety and teaches people how to take ownership and solve problems themselves.

Chapter 7

Sustaining Commitment— A *Roadmap*

Chapter Outline

SO, HOW DO YOU SUSTAIN COMMITMENT, ONCE YOU ACHIEVE IT?

Succinctly and repetitively make the case for ownership, using the influence techniques outlined in Chapter 5—How to Influence Commitment. Your efforts should compel people to own and commit to the changes, and also clearly show them how to make the expected changes.

You must also ensure that the expectations for change are aligned with, and fully integrated into, communication, education, and training. Measure performance, compliance, and all targeted impacts for the change. Then, reward commitment, address noncompliance, and coach people to a higher level of commitment. Remember, that these are the "glue" between the puzzle pieces, that were discussed in detail in Section I about culture. (See steps IV, V, and VI of the *Roadmap* for culture, as they are the same steps to building commitment.)

Food Safety. DOI: http://dx.doi.org/10.1016/B978-0-12-811189-5.00007-6

In Section II, we more specifically outline the tools you can use to build commitment across your organization, demonstrating the importance of that commitment to new and existing employees.

Now, let's look first at the means by which you can communicate expectations to new and existing employees.

MAKE SURE EMPLOYEE EDUCATION AND TRAINING EMPHASIZES FOOD SAFETY, FROM THE START...

Onboarding or employee orientation is the best way to orient a new employee or manager about what is important to know about the company from the start. Food Safety and its importance should be covered with employees as soon as they start. This should not just be a paragraph of information that is often lost in the rest of the onboarding material. It should be prominent, well-thought-out information that not only emphasizes the importance of Food Safety, but also describes what they need to do in the company, every day. Information should outline company standards and include specific requirements in their job to ensure Food Safety.

Another best practice is to offer half-day culture refresher workshops, taught by executives. If an organization requires one or two of these per year, per employee, the education and training can highlight the integration of Food Safety into the day-to-day work.

Education and training can also occur during short discussions to review problems that have arisen and develop solutions. Reinforcement through short, interactive sessions is a valuable tool.

If the organization doesn't offer ongoing education and training options, the same content can be incorporated into the education and training available to people based on their position. It is good practice for any organization to plan for the education and training of their employees and to track people's progress through that learning cycle. Doing so provides another opportunity to reinforce the need for commitment to Food Safety initiatives. Additionally, departmental training will ensure a unified understanding and effort toward Food Safety. At the same time departmental teams will develop a common understanding of its importance.

If managers in your organization are struggling to manage performance, recognize good performance, or correct unacceptable performance, they may also need training. This involves holding tougher conversations. They may need leadership training in conflict management and performance management. Once expectations are set, communicated, trained, and measured, it rests with the employee's supervisor to be sure behavior has aligned with expectations. People who do not change may need further assistance. People who cannot master that change after further help and/or who choose not to comply should not be allowed to stay with the organization.

DEVELOP INTERNAL COLLATERAL TO EMPHASIZE FOOD SAFETY

Brand the commitment to Food Safety and refer to it everywhere you can. In your break room, on the walls of your hallways, on the outside of steps that people take, on the inside of elevators, even in your parking lot. Reinforce the message of the commitment, so that people don't forget it. Include it in the salutations of your executive's e-mail signatures, and put it on any intranet/internal digital displays available to you.

If you regularly communicate with your employees in a newsletter, include articles about success stories. Show them how Food Safety can and has positively impacted their jobs and their company. People want to take pride in what they are doing but also want to know how they benefit from what they are doing correctly. Change the message up, keep it fresh, issue new reminders so that this does not just become something they ignore. Make it interesting.

OFFER JOB-DESCRIPTION-BASED PERFORMANCE REVIEWS

All positions within a company should have written Job Descriptions. A Job Description that is specific to the job is the main way of communicating expectations. While many companies use other documents to communicate expectations, such as Key Performance Indices (KPI's) budgets, annual goals, or departmental expectations, the Job Description should incorporate *all* expectations. Most organizations do not have very solid Job Descriptions. They are usually done too quickly and many contain the same language when the job is really not the same. Job Descriptions should clearly outline which tasks within a process the position is responsible to achieve. It should also include result and goal expectations of that position. Finally, the Job Description should include a thorough list of skills necessary for a person to accomplish the tasks and meet the results. As appropriate, Food Safety and the requirements of that position to support it should be clear. Without Job Descriptions, there is not a consistent agreement as to what work a person is responsible for in his/her position. Job Descriptions with specific tasks, results, and skills needed for the job are likely to allow an organization to hire people better and to get better results from their existing team.

Performance Reviews should measure the effective completion of job expectations. The use of generic Performance Reviews will generally not get you what you are looking for. If that is what your company uses, work with Human Resources to influence consideration of a more job-specific review system. That change could take some time, so in the meantime, work with them to adjust the generic measures so Food Safety and the behaviors associated with it are prominent in the review.

Job Descriptions and Performance Reviews should define expectations and evaluate the person's behavior and commitment to Food Safety. The verbiage could read something like:

- "Employee understands and consistently adheres to policies and procedures defined within the Food Safety Policy." There should be an even more detailed Job Description for those employees whose job this encompasses.

For the employees that also manage others (supervisors, managers, leaders) their Job Description and Performance Review should include:

- "Supervisor/manager/leader sets a solid example in Food Safety by consistently adhering to policies and procedures defined within the Food Safety Policy."

- "Supervisor/manager/leader holds his/her employees accountable for consistently adhering to policies and procedures defined within the Food Safety Policy, and effectively deals with adherence if it is not acceptable."
- "Supervisor/manager/leader rewards and recognizes employees for consistently adhering to policies and procedures defined within the Food Safety Policy."
- "Supervisor/manager/leader regularly includes Food Safety in education, training, and communication."
- "Supervisor/manager/leader contributes to the continuous improvement of Food Safety processes."

The best approach is to develop specific Job Descriptions and related Performance Reviews that fully capture the expectations and the result goals or performance metrics of that employee's job, to support the right steps to address Food Safety. This approach actually links the review to the Job Descriptions. Both reflect expectations, tasks, and goals within the job and emphasize those that support Food Safety. When using this approach, the employee knows the expectations of his/her job, the tasks he/she is responsible for to meet those expectations and the results that are impacted by his/her work. Then, performance is measured upon it and directly connected to the employee meeting the expectations required.

REVIEW METRICS, REGULARLY

Determine how you will know if commitment is solid and develop a scorecard that regularly shows movement on the hard numbers. You may need to work with your Finance Department to develop the scorecard. Visibility should be daily if possible, but never less frequently than monthly.

Finally, develop a checklist for the soft numbers so that you can check improvement. Run through that checklist at the beginning of each week or month to see if you are seeing improvement. Talk about improvement or the lack of it, often and openly.

ONCE AGAIN, THE "GLUE"

Remember that a Food Safety program cannot be implemented without solid levels of management commitment that cross all departments. The absence of such commitment and lack of real departmental cooperation will result in one of three scenarios in which the desired outcome is *not* reached:

- Nothing is done to advance the efforts (inactivity).
- People begin to talk about it, but don't really do anything differently (lip service).
- People try to do positive things, but stop because it is too hard or they are penalized instead of rewarded (misalignment).

For Food Safety to develop, evolve, improve, and be successfully implemented within your organization, your leaders must openly commit to it as a priority in words and action. They must gain similar commitments from all of their people.

To make commitment visible to the organization in ways that impact change in culture, structure, and actions, leaders must use the "glue":

- Communication/education and training
- Metrics to measure success
- Accountability for change
- Influence/persuasion

Section III

The Impact of Organizational Structure on Food Safety

Chapter 8

Fundamentals of Organizational Structure Irrespective of Industry

Chapter Outline

So, you want to get more serious about Food Safety, but how do you make decisions regarding structure to ensure you are able to meet your goals? The objective for any organization developing a structure to support Food Safety is to make decisions that enable an effective technical organization. In order to do that, one must understand the organizational dynamics inherent in structure. This will allow for good decisions with respect to how the work and positions should be structured.

PROCESS FIRST

All too often, organizational change happens because the leaders at the top think the work is not being done as well as it should be. For decades, an "organizational re-structure" has been touted as a means to greater productivity and improved process. Often, re-structuring has yielded less than adequate results, sometimes even reversing company objectives. This is most often caused by quick decisions made without looking at all the considerations.

Many companies, when tackling organizational structure, try to re-invent a structure using a "pencil and box" activity with a few

Food Safety. DOI: http://dx.doi.org/10.1016/B978-0-12-811189-5.00008-8
79

people in a room determining if they think the person they penciled into a box can handle the objectives noted for that position. This is a big mistake. Instead, they should identify the process behind the necessary workflow and map all tasks to jobs. In that way, it becomes very clear what the position should be accomplishing. Only after this occurs, can the leaders involved in the exercise make an informed decision about who can handle the work and who should oversee it. This also lays the foundation to write a much better Job Description. Be sure to involve enough people so that you have a thorough knowledge of the workflow.

Structure is the way an organization is built to complete the desired work. It encompasses who reports to whom, but also how the work is structured within a position. Every task within a process should reside in someone's job. That person must clearly understand that the task is their responsibility and exactly how it should be done. That person should be held accountable for the thorough and effective completion of that task. They should fully understand how that task fits into the process so they can effectively connect it with the rest of the work. This will enable clear hand-offs between people/departments who own different parts of the process.

STRUCTURE CONSIDERATIONS: GROUND RULES

- Indirect (dotted line) reporting relationships rarely work!—The direct supervisor generally has the say and his/her goals will take precedence. Indirect reporting relationships are put into place to make the indirect supervisor feel as though they are guiding the work. The indirect supervisor's input into the work goals and performance can be helpful, but they rarely have any authority. The one exception to this in a Food Safety structure is if the Food Safety Department reports to the CEO or COO. This can illustrate the importance the organization places on Food Safety. When the "C"-level is involved, they likely will have authority.
  - Give the work to the position most connected to the goal outcome. Teach influence skills to enable connectivity from other parties.

- Dual reporting relationships do not work!—Work has to have one person responsible for its completion for effective accountability. When an employee reports to two different people directly, he/she will spend more time trying to balance the objectives between the two bosses than actually doing the work. In the rare instances where two supervisors of the same person actually agree upon work objectives and/or have connected goals, the communication styles are different enough for the employee to often be confused and feel their role is to run interference so they can accommodate those differences. In any situation, work is more political than actual.
  - Give the work to the position most connected to the desired goals outcome. Teach influence skills to enable connectivity with other parties.

- Organizational decisions should be functional rather than personal—The right organizational structure should never be dependent upon the people in the role. While you definitely need to take great care in placing the right person in the role, with the correct skills to do the job, you must set the structure up to accommodate change in personalities. Be sure there is not a conflict of interest or goals when making decisions regarding who will manage a certain function within a structure.
  - For example, if Dan, a Food Safety Manager reports to Jane, who oversees Operations, and Jane's and Dan's goals are in some conflict, it can only work if Dan can stand up to Jane. If Dan leaves and the next person will not stand up to Jane, the structure will not work.

- Goals alignment is critical—The supervisor of a position should have the same goals as the position he/she manages. If the goals are in conflict, or out of sync, they will not be met. There should be mutual success by both parties/teams if the goals are met. One should not cancel out the other.
  - For example, if Jill is a Grocery Supervisor in a Grocery Store and Jake is the Perishable Supervisor, each is accountable for in-store sales of their categories. If Jill is expected to have 55% of the revenue mix and Jake is expected to have 58% of the revenue mix, there is no possible way they

can make their goals together. If they are running the store together, the competition will be counter-productive.

- o In another example, Stan is the COO and he is incented on productivity, but he manages Dayna who is the Food Safety Manager. She is incented on quality. Better quality may, in fact, reduce the baseline of productivity to which the organization has become accustomed. To address this situation, Dayna for example should demonstrate to Stan how a strong Food Safety System can actually enhance productivity by having less rejected product.
- Placement in the organizational hierarchy sends a strong message as to how important a particular initiative is to the organization.
- When configuring structure, pay attention to the numbers.
  - o A leader should never directly manage more than eight (8) Direct Reports. Five to seven is preferable. This enables the leader to adequately develop, lead, and manage the work. In some cases, where a leader is managing a group of people that are, for the most part, high performing and do the same type of work, a leader can handle up to 12. This is not the case if each person in the role needs something different for their growth and development.
  - o Conversely, a one-on-one, or one-on-two relationship is too narrow of a scope for a leader. While this may be a good ratio for a new manager to let them learn leadership skills, most leaders can and should do more. Evaluate a one-on-one hierarchy to see if both positions are truly needed.

STRUCTURE CHANGE—A ROADMAP

As a result, structure change should always encompass:

- What work actually needs to be completed? Define the process in place and/or needed process change when forming structure. The steps allocated to a certain position should be included in all Job Descriptions and Performance Reviews.
- What results are actually necessary from the work? Set clear expectations. These will be used in communication, education,

and training. They should be present in the Job Description, expectations, and Performance Review process.

- What skills are necessary to complete the work? Identify competencies needed by the person in the position to effectively complete the work allocated to the position.
- Who should oversee/lead the work? Give the work to the position most connected to the goals outcome.
- How is the team incented? Be sure to align goals, so that the leader of an area has goals that are in alignment with the teams he/she oversees.
- Once decided, develop clear Job Description and expectation documents to support the change.
- Once finalized, develop an effective Change Communication Plan to steer the organization to realize the benefits planned for the structure change. Be sure to include planning for the communication of job change to impacted individuals. Be sure to include education and training.

Following these rules and starting with a good understanding of the desired process will ensure that the people in place can better meet the desired goals.

Chapter 9

Food Safety Organizational Structures Within Types of Companies

Chapter Outline

THE MUST-HAVES

There are infinite ways to build a structure to support goals. As we move into the exploration of delivering Food Safety goals within different structures, you will want to keep one thing in mind. Be sure that the Food Safety Department (and any related Quality positions) report to a position high enough in the organization that they have access to present ideas for consideration to a decision maker. Food Safety must be in a structure in which they can be heard.

Depending on the size of the company, the Food Safety Department may be one person handling Food Safety, as a Food Safety Coordinator or Manager, or there may be multiple people reporting to a Food Safety Lead who is titled as a Manager, Director, or VP of Food Safety or Technical Services. If there are

Food Safety. DOI: http://dx.doi.org/10.1016/B978-0-12-811189-5.00009-X

multiple people in the department, the Job Descriptions for each member of the Food Safety Department should specifically outline responsibilities for each position. For purposes of this discussion, we will refer to the position that directly manages the Food Safety Department (regardless of size) as the Food Safety Department Head.

It is possible that the Food Safety Department Head is a member of the (top-level) Executive Leadership Team and reports to a C-level position. If not, the Food Safety Department Head should be supervised by a member of the Executive Leadership Team who supports and cares about Food Safety and who is incented with Food Safety goals. We will refer to this position as the Key Leader Overseeing Food Safety. He/she should have access to, or be, a key decision maker. This person should clearly outline the required commitment to Food Safety and its goals within the organization, as should any other documents that outline goals (ie, KPIs, goals, process documentation, etc.). The Job Description should also clearly outline the responsibility this person has to review and make Food Safety decisions. Selection for the position should be made with that in mind.

Together the Food Safety Department Head and the Key Leader Overseeing Food Safety should be held responsible for interacting with and influencing multiple departments as solutions are identified and developed. Therefore, this should be a job requirement for all involved. People with good skills in this area should be hired to hold those positions. All employees within this structure should seek out further development in influencing decisions.

Note that we are *not necessarily advocating* that Food Safety *must* report to a senior-level leader in the organization. While that may make the most sense for your organization, and it certainly sends a strong message as to the importance of Food Safety; the efforts can be successful even if positioned within the structure at a lower level. So, if you are reading this and currently report to a lower level in the organization, it can work. Success will rely heavily on the ability of the Food Safety team to build respect, and the Food Safety Department Head to build respect and influence across the organization. Remember that Food Safety cannot be seen as being compromised.

WHAT DEPARTMENT?

There is not one best answer as to where Food Safety should reside, or if it should be its own department. The places where most Food Safety reside other than reporting directly to the CEO or COO are Operations, Research & Development (R&D), Technical Services, or Legal. The following table takes a look at some of the advantages and disadvantages.

Department	Advantages	Disadvantages
Operations	Operations is driving Production and Food Safety must be fully integrated into the production process. Both the Food Safety Department and competent, responsible operators can truly benefit from learning to understand each other.	It is very easy for goals to be conflicting. Typically Operations is responsible for getting things out the door fast and cheap. If your organization pits Food Safety against Operations, this is not the best place to start.
	Be sure to align Food Safety goals into the goal set for Operations. Be sure to have people in roles that are collaborative and not adversarial.	
Research and Development (R&D) and/ or Product Development (PD)	They talk each other's language and understand each other's concerns. Food Safety, R&D, and PD, employ highly technical people.	They may not challenge each other to build the necessary skills for communication and influence. They may not interact as well across the organization. They may have different goals.
	Be sure to provide ongoing training for these teams to build respect and influence across the organization and between each other.	

Department	Advantages	Disadvantages
Technical Services	This area may have Food Safety, Regulatory, R&D, and Quality reporting to it. This helps to foster intra-departmental cooperation since the goals of the each group can be aligned and conflicts quickly addressed for resolution.	The leader of this group must establish his/ her competency to the organization and understand the company's overall business initiatives, as well as goals, in order to be successful.

Be sure the Technical Services leader understands each of the areas for which they are responsible and how to forge partnerships with other department leaders.

Legal	Legal has a high sense of urgency about minimizing risk, which is the sole purpose of Food Safety. Not only are their goals aligned, but their missions are also interdependent.	Legal can often have more of a stiff-arm approach to telling the organization they have to do something, rather than building the organization's commitment to the reasons behind taking the appropriate steps.

Be sure to position Legal as a partner in building organizational commitment

There are other places Food Safety can reside, depending on the type of company. It may reside in Quality Assurance (QA), particularly for transportation or if the company also does non-food products. Food Safety is, in part, a QA function, so putting it in a structure as an element of QA is only applicable if there is other QA oversight. It may reside in merchandising, particularly for retailers. It may reside in Service, particularly for hospitality. It may reside in Product Development, although that is often related to R&D. Finally, it may reside in Purchasing, particularly if the company is sourcing ingredients from other providers who must also meet Food Safety guidelines and standards.

There is not a best answer across the board, so evaluate your organization's needs for the best answer to bridge the gap from where you are currently, to where you need to be operating for the longer term. Remember that goals must be aligned between Food Safety and the department in which it resides. Also, know that both sets of goals, while aligned, must also reside in the organization's strategic business plan as a prominent initiative that gets talked about, often. *If you put Food Safety in everyone's performance measures, this will ensure a much greater level of success.*

If the top Food Safety "practitioner" in a company works for someone who is constantly challenging basic Food Safety premises and not supporting programs or decisions, this will become frustrating. Eventually the "battle of wills" can lead to an absence of understanding, which can lead to a catastrophic event for the organization. In order to avoid this, everyone involved should connect business needs to Food Safety needs in order to begin collaborative dialog.

OTHER ORGANIZATIONAL STRUCTURE CONSIDERATIONS: FOOD SAFETY

- Do everything possible to avoid silos when building a structure to support Food Safety.
- Look at the full integration of related departments (R&D, Supply Chain Operations, and Food Safety) their goals, business planning, and processes.
- Good QA helps to develop guidelines and provides education and training. They enable tools for the job and check for compliance. Be sure the structure clearly outlines who does each part of this and that process clearly maps how the work should be done. Most often, this is a Food Safety function.
- Good Quality Control (QC) often resides in Operations and is the way an organization ensures that guidelines are followed and product is made consistently and safely. As a result, the best structure pairs the efforts of Food Safety and QA with QC. Both parties should participate in customizing the guidelines to their particular situation.

CONSIDERATIONS BY TYPE OF COMPANY

The chart below identifies some additional considerations based on the type of corporate structure your company has.

Single Entity—Centralized

Definition and Structure	Challenges	Solutions
Classic corporate structure with oversight on all local execution or implementation. Most often, leadership levels are flatter with a vertical reporting structure that makes decisions centrally and communicates them. Food Safety should report up, as high up as possible.	Food Safety is often seen as an overhead cost. They are not seen as connected to the business. There is often a different view of practice (what is actually done) versus science (what should be done) that can hinder successful efforts.	Food Safety should be as integrated as possible to the direction being developed at a centralized level. Food Safety professionals will need to work hard to demonstrate their ability to understand and connect to the business. They should be careful not to "over-science" and to demonstrate practical responsibility.

Single Entity—De-Centralized or Franchised

Definition and Structure	Challenges	Solutions
Classic corporate structure with little oversight on all local execution or implementation. In the case of a franchise, corporate may only provide standards, guidelines, and branding, transferring full responsibility for local execution to the local teams. Most often, leadership levels are transferred to the local level with a business support located at corporate headquarters. While the single entity and the franchise are separate legal structures, they face some of the same challenges in ensuring Food Safety.	Food Safety can be lost in the focus of the team at the local level. Local leadership may see and understand the need for Food Safety, but may not build the culture within their business unit to support it. They may not allocate resources to oversight.	Food Safety should be as integrated as possible to the standards being set. Food Safety should have a presence in the corporate structure. Food Safety should be mandatory for local teams. Thus, the Food Safety department at an organization like this will need to focus on education and training, developing tools for easy execution, creating metrics for the team leader to utilize. They may also maintain a compliance responsibility. Internal audits may be necessary.

Privately held companies have less shareholder expectations and often serve a much smaller set of goals. They frequently have family stakeholders and decisions are often subject to family dynamics. Some will openly share metrics while others will not. Public companies drive shareholder value and have infinitely more shareholders. They will value access to numbers, goals, and their related metrics, and disclosure is required.

Multiple Entity—More than One Business Department or Company Reporting into Corporate or Parent Oversight

Definition and Structure	Challenges	Solutions
Multiple entities reside under one umbrella. Structures can vary widely. Corporate goals and standards are usually fed down to the multiple entities. These are usually public.	Everything that happens within a multiple entity structure is built to support the top-tier standards and goals. This will present challenges if the standards and goals have not encompassed Food Safety.	Since everything that happens within a multiple entity structure is built to support standards and goals, the best approach is to offer solid processes, with effective education and training to each entity. Each entity should have a person with Food Safety compliance responsibility.

Mergers and Acquisitions

A word about mergers and acquisitions. They will create or add to the complexity of a multiple entity structure.

If the acquisition is done with the intention of integration, the corporate entity should have a strong team to assess the needs for integration. Integration itself should include careful process analysis, intentional position and structure design along with strong education and training to ensure a smooth cultural transition.

If the acquisition is done with the intention of leaving the acquired entity independent, the acquiring organization's Food Safety presence should still provide standards and guidelines, provide education and training to meet those, and be sure someone is measuring compliance. The acquiring organization may also look at metrics to ensure culture development. There is a chance that this type of acquisition is an investment for short term payout and that the acquiring organization does not have a commitment to Food Safety, or a presence within its structure to deal with it. In this case, the acquiring organization has a moral and legal responsibility to turn out safe food, even if the team is incented on fast, cheap delivery of product and/or rapid revenue growth.

Global Considerations

US-owned, international companies may find that Food Safety is in the domestic corporate entity but not as strong in the international business units. The Food Safety in the domestic entity must work to understand the imperatives in other countries. Different countries have different acceptable standards. For example, if a company considers personal hygiene differently, they will not easily see how their standards impact the output of the product, negatively.

Internationally owned US companies must develop ways of measuring and communicating to bridge the gap between what must be done in the United States and communicate the needs with cultural sensitivities.

Global partnerships should be done with a mutual understanding of means and methods of doing business. They should understand the financials, goals, and risk tolerance.

CONCLUSION

If an organization is doing well and growing, Food Safety can help them by strengthening brand and customer/consumer satisfaction. Partner with Marketing and Sales to leverage this advantage.

A business simply cannot engage in practices that will put Food Safety at risk, no matter how it is structured, as a corporation. A business simply cannot engage in a "look the other way" mentality about Food Safety, which leads to inactivity that puts their customers, consumers, and futures at risk.

While the bottom line is often viewed as the "bottom line" for what is done at a company, without an adequate Food Safety commitment, be it people, money, or departmental cooperation, the company will put itself at an unacceptable risk.

Section IV

Implementation — The *Roadmap*

Chapter 10

Connecting the Puzzle Pieces to Develop Your *Roadmap*

Chapter Outline

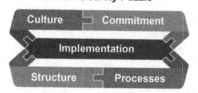

The Food Safety Puzzle™

So far, this book has outlined several things for the reader about several pieces of the puzzle. In the Introduction, we talked about processes and procedures regarding Food Safety. The guidelines for Food Safety are backed with processes and procedures that are well documented, well known and, most often, regulated. This book was not written to help people identify what processes and procedures to follow to ensure effective Food Safety practices, but rather how to get people to follow those processes and procedures.

- In Section I, Chapter 1 "What Is *Effective* Food Safety Culture?," we dealt with the methodology to change, enhance, or shape culture.

Food Safety. DOI: http://dx.doi.org/10.1016/B978-0-12-811189-5.00010-6

- In Chapter 2 "What Gets in the Way? Barriers and Solutions," we explored barriers to culture change, offering an understanding of the barrier, its cause, and potential solutions.
- In Chapter 3 "How Does Culture Come to Be? A *Roadmap*," we offered a *Roadmap to Culture Change*. This was the first of our *Roadmaps*, and is a six-step, easy to follow methodology to ensure cultural change. It is a good place to start, because the six steps also lay the groundwork to build Organizational and Management Commitment. The six steps are:

   1. Plan
   2. Dialog
   3. Change Process
   4. Communicate Change
   5. Develop Success Measures
   6. Implement and Hold Accountable

   In other words, decide what to do (steps 1, 2, and 3), tell people you are going to do it (step 4), show them how to do it (step 4), and be sure everyone is doing what you ask (step 5). Celebrate success (step 6), and move substandard performance to a higher level (step 6).

- In Chapter 4 "What Can You Do? Your Role and Its Impact on Positive Culture Change," we offered practical application advice to allow you to assess the type of culture you have in your company, determine what you can do, based on your role and type of culture your team is experiencing, to follow the six-step *Roadmap to Culture Change*.

The main premise for Section I offered a way to fully embrace Food Safety in your organization by elevating the Food Safety initiative to a high level within the Strategic Business Plan. You must then make sure you put into motion all the elements that support change of day-to-day work and make sure it is happening. Once in motion, you have identified all the components you need to direct organizational commitment. You will notice that 3 of the 4 "glue" elements (see next Chapter 11) are woven throughout this six-step Roadmap to Culture Change: Communication/ Education and Training (step 4); Metrics to Measure Success (step 5); and Accountability for Change (step 6).

- In Section II, Chapter 5—How to Influence Commitment, we introduced a methodology to build your influence skills as a member of your organization. Remember that influence is a "glue" element. Influence is the only way to get organizational or management commitment, but it is dependent upon the work done in the six-step *Roadmap to Culture Change.* Remember that commitment and culture are intertwined. Commitment is a critical ingredient to create culture, but culture cannot sustain itself without commitment. Also, commitment cannot sustain itself in the absence of a supporting culture. This chapter explored differences in goals, how we view risk and how we communicate, in general. Remember to keep interactions proactive, positive, and productive. Stay practical and show others how you can help them meet their goals. The objective is to build "owners" of Food Safety by speaking their language and understanding the metrics that drive their behaviors.
- Chapter 6 "How to Measure Commitment" dealt with Measures. There is the "glue" again-metrics. We explained several ways to be sure that work that needs to be done is being done.
- In Chapter 7 "Sustaining Commitment—A *Roadmap*," we offered the second of our *Roadmaps.* This *Roadmap* is not a set of steps, but rather a checklist of the things that must support commitment in order for it to continue to be relevant. Notice they are all connected as "glue" elements.
  - ○ Employee education and training should emphasize Food Safety, from the start. It should also be part of continual reinforcement activities.
  - ○ Internal collateral material for organizational communication should emphasize Food Safety.
  - ○ Job Descriptions should emphasize Food Safety. They should be the driver for Performance Reviews so that the employees are evaluated on how well they deliver on Food Safety.
  - ○ Metrics should indicate compliance and should be reviewed regularly.
- In Section III, Chapter 8 "Fundamentals of Organizational Structure Irrespective of Industry," we outlined several considerations when looking at structure within your organization.

- Chapter 9 "Food Safety Organizational Structures Within Types of Companies" took an in-depth look at structural considerations when making decisions about where Food Safety should report and how it should be integrated into the company. There are no "right" answers, but rather several things to consider.

A *ROADMAP* TO DEVELOP AN IMPLEMENTATION PLAN

In this, Section IV, Chapter 10 "Connecting the Puzzle Pieces to Develop Your *Roadmap*," we show how the puzzle pieces actually come together. Implementation is what you need to do to make it all come together. The best way to implement is to be sure that Food Safety is a focal point and imperative within all of your business practices. Always start with the planning process. If your organization already plans effectively, be sure Food Safety is a prominent part of that planning. If your organization does not regularly plan, use this initiative to get them started. Remember that to effectively make progress toward improving Food Safety in your company, you have to be realistic about what you need to change. Thus, the following steps define a *Roadmap* for developing your Implementation Plan.

1. First, define your current reality. Ask, "Where are we?"
2. Then, determine future objectives. Ask, "Where should we be?"
3. Next, determine what is missing? Know your challenges and problems.
4. Then, determine what is needed to get to where you should be. Identify and develop effective solutions.
5. Finally, develop your Implementation Plan.

Fully understand what is happening today. Organizations often don't see their opportunities. Seek objective feedback and ask the people doing the work what is going on, ensuring that you are open to feedback. Productive dialog requires that communication flows up, down, and across the entire organization. This is how you should start this work. This interactive dialog should become a way of life. Leaders in an organization need to know what is really happening, all the time.

Identify a comprehensive series of guidelines. Know exactly what practices you want to exist in your organization. Understand your goals to implement Food Safety practices to prevent mistakes, keep problems from occurring and be able to effectively respond to issues. This work should be collaborative and involve all key leaders—who should be getting input from their teams.

Determine what needs to change. The success of this step depends fully on the accuracy of steps 1 and 2. To understand what is missing, you have to know where you are and where you are going. Once the team knows these two things, the missing parts (and their root causes) become very clear. We call this the Gap. Your objective is to bridge the Gap between where you are today and what you want to and will achieve tomorrow.

Determine how to change what is currently taking place. This will involve process analysis and your process change planning. In a culture of continual process improvement, this will happen more easily. In a culture that still thinks of that thing you changed 5 years ago as new, this will take more effort. The objective is to provide specific guidance to all levels about solutions that effectively improve something in the business. This work should also address the need to remove the causes that exist of the undesirable situations (i.e., root cause solutions).

Once you have completed this work, you have the foundation for the Implementation Plan. Then, you can develop a detailed plan for implementation of the changes necessary to focus on Food Safety. Identify the details of the solutions. Fully outline what needs to be accomplished, how it should be accomplished, when and by whom. Some of the components of this plan will be one-time initiatives, whereas others will be ongoing. Most of these solutions will be embedded in the process, which will prompt overall process change. Remember to look at efficiency within processes when adjusting or changing them. Good processes need to be based upon best practices (owned by all) rather than tribal knowledge (owned by each individual). Documentation is paramount in this step. Details are a critical part of any change. It is easy to talk about what to do, but not as easy to determine how to do it. Until that detail work is done, people will not be able to do what you are asking them to do. It is trite but true that "the devil is in the details".

A Few Words About Plans

Most businesses do some type of planning. Most leaders think it is strategic. All too often plans are not long term and are not collaborative across the organization. Food Safety is best embraced if it is a part of a Strategic Business Planning process.

WHAT IS STRATEGIC BUSINESS PLANNING?

In its purest form, "strategy" is the means by which an organization determines what they want to accomplish. A plan encompasses the way an organization wishes to achieve it. Therefore, a truly "strategic plan" aligns the actions of today with the goals of tomorrow. It is long-term, future-oriented, and clearly outlines what needs to occur to reach the organization's goals. In short, good strategy improves business results. The main reason to proceed with the process of developing a solid strategy is to grow profits leading to an organization's substantial growth and/or sustainable recovery.

Some forms of planning commonly needed within an organization may be confused with Strategic Business Planning.

"Project Planning" is used by a project manager to determine exactly how that project gets completed. He/she thinks through objectives for the work, who should do it, when it should be done and the necessary communication. Thus, projects within an organization become a key means of achieving strategy, but project managers should always be sure that the projects are connecting to and supporting strategic goals. Project planning, when done in isolation, generates work activity but may not always produce results. This type of planning is generally done by most people in the organization in order to drive work completion. A Strategic Business Plan must have an accompanying Implementation Plan, which will include detailed Project Planning.

"Annual Goals Planning" is often used by leaders of a company to articulate to others what needs to be done within a given year. Usually, goals are assigned and added to the performance management. Quite often, the goals are financial. It is common to meet with C-level leaders about strategy who indicate that they have a good strategic plan, but, upon closer review, it is shorter-term, more narrowly focused, and not likely to be directed toward the organization's end-game. Calling a plan a strategic plan does not make it one.

"Business Planning" is the way leaders of a company or entrepreneurs starting a company can plan the path they intend to grow revenues and reach financial goals. A formalized business plan is generally required to attract investors or convince a board of directors to make a change. It includes several elements also included in a good Strategic Business Plan. For example, it calls for financial projections, market analysis, and a sales plan. It is most often intermediate in focus. All of these elements should be included in strategic business planning and, if not developed, the strategic business planning discussions should address them. The key difference between a "Business Plan" and a "Strategic Business Plan" is both the process by which they are developed as well as the execution levels contained in the Strategic Business Plan's accompanying Implementation Plan. This is generally not present in a Business Plan.

"Budget Planning" is the organization's means of developing financial metrics. If a company drives strategy from their budget planning, they run the risk of not being able to meet the goals as there is not an identified path from one to the other.

In the Chapter 11 , we will address the Change Communication Plan and the Metrics Plan, which should also be a part of the Strategic Business Plan. We will also address how to sustain the effort through accountability.

Chapter 11

Some Concluding Words About the "Glue"

Chapter Outline

All Strategic Business Plans must have a detailed Implementation Plan with a solid path to communicate the change and to measure its success. Remember, that the "glue" includes:

- communication/education/training—tell them; show them;
- metrics to measure success—check them;
- accountability for change—reward success; address failure/noncompliance;
- influence everyone as often as possible.

In order to implement your *Change Communication Plan*, it should be detailed and comprehensive. You should determine who needs to know what? Tell people what and why, and show them how.

Develop a detailed plan for communication to support your change. You are changing the rules of the game, so inform the players. This will involve communication to everyone. Tell everyone in every way possible. Employees directly impacted, or from those whom major change will be required, should be told individually.

This requires education for those doing or supporting the change, to give them the needed information to understand why the change is occurring and what it means for them.

Finally, training should be done for those needing to change what they actually do. This should involve training in process

Food Safety. DOI: http://dx.doi.org/10.1016/B978-0-12-811189-5.00011-8

and skills while also offering opportunities for guided practice. Documentation of the new process can be used to train employees.

Employee Job Descriptions should be changed to reflect exactly what they are responsible for accomplishing. Process and procedure manuals should be updated for clear references during and after training. For each involved party, clearly define and demonstrate what they will be doing differently.

Your *Metrics Plan* should tell you if the targeted changes are happening. You should determine how you know it is successful. Develop appropriate metrics. Once guidelines have been set, defined, and communicated, they must be measured across the organization, within departments and for each employee. Remember that measurement drives behavior, so don't measure anything that doesn't tell you how you are doing, compared with your goal. Test and validate your methods to be sure you are on target. This is generally more effective when utilizing systems that can generate progress reports.

HOW DO WE CONTINUE TO IMPROVE?

Once you measure, be sure to reward and recognize success or desired behaviors as often as possible, no matter how small. This will remind others to follow the same patterns while keeping the targets on the forefront. Also, if someone is not meeting expectations, leaders need to hold them accountable for aligning their behavior with what is expected. Remember that failure to address missed expectations will send a strong message that it is OK. This will impede any attempts at improvement within organizational culture. The ability to ensure accountability and appropriate reward will be enhanced if leaders can rely on a system to remind them about following up, tracking progress, and checkpoints. They also need to have good skills for follow-through, influence, and conflict management.

Anything you try to do within your organization requires the "glue" to be fully successful. That is why you have seen these four things in every section. They are organizational staples for effectiveness.

If your organization is embarking on the commitment to Food Safety, use these *Roadmaps* to make sure that your efforts are both comprehensive and successful.

If you are in a key leadership position, use this information as a means to engage others in dialog about the implementation of the effort. If your organization needs to make this commitment but you are not a member of the key leadership team, use this information as a foundation to engage in dialog influencing others to commit to such efforts.

Develop the ability to influence and communicate in terms that management understands. Remember that numbers talk to people. Arm yourself with an understanding of pertinent numbers for your organization and take some time to understand what has happened to organizations that did not do this.

Finally, if Food Safety is your job in an organization, be thorough about the details.

Think of Food Safety precaution as if it were a type of insurance. Individuals buy insurance to transfer risk and gain peace of mind by making the decision to protect themselves from catastrophe. When your organization commits to increasing quality standards to ensure Food Safety, the changes must become routine and daily to be sustainable.

Like any other Strategic Initiative, it won't happen without an action plan that tells each person involved what he/she should do, how to do it, and why. You must also provide employees with the tools to do what you are asking them to do. Tools include financial resources, people, equipment, education, training, and departmental cooperation.

Remember that Food Safety needs to be your top priority, not an afterthought. It is far less costly if you implement Food Safety practices before you have an incident. If someone finds something in your food, or if he or she gets sick (or dies) because of something in your food, life as you know it today will forever change.

Remember that the best way to be as safe as you need to be is to ask yourself a very simple question, "would you feed the product to your children".

Appendix A

A Few Other Things That May Be Useful...

Note that these segments include information from EDGES'
Whitepaper series.

As a Food Safety professional, you are tasked with knowing what your organization does, knowing what it should do to deliver safe food products, and influencing people in your organization of the importance of Food Safety. Without this influence, your organization will not be committed to making the necessary and sustained changes for an effective Food Safety program. Many of the things that foster good Food Safety are part of bigger systems that may already exist in a company. Any strong, quality-oriented organization should already be doing them. If your organization is doing these things, you can fit in what needs to be done regarding Food Safety quite easily by working with the owners of the system(s). If your organization is not doing these things, they should be. Your job will be more difficult. You will actually have to influence leaders to make a commitment to a system that is broader than Food Safety but that will support Food Safety.

The premise of this book is to approach Food Safety as a Strategic Initiative or Imperative. Within the body of the book, we dealt with ways to influence these Strategic Initiatives, beginning with ways to get your organization to see the need for this type of planning if they do not do it now or if planning is not a discipline in your company. We then outlined steps to incorporate Food Safety into the planning process to be sure it gets the prominence and attention it needs to be successful. We also addressed other key tools. The direction we gave you assumes that some planning process exists in your organization, but it may not. This section is designed to provide you with information that you can share with decision-makers regarding these larger systems to encourage them to develop the systems to use for the overall company and to include Food Safety. Your advantage will be that establishing an effective planning system helps everything the organization tries to do, not just Food Safety. The goal is to get others who will benefit to help you influence the development and adoption of all or some of these systems.

Examples of these systems include:

- Strong *Process Documentation Systems* to define and document needed changes and current practices
- Strong *Corporate Communication Systems* to support change using various methods of communicating
- *Job Description-Based Performance Review Systems* that hold people accountable for the desired changes
- *A Model for Process Change.*

Now let's look at these examples in more detail.

PROCESS DOCUMENTATION SYSTEMS

Process documentation systems enable the organization to clearly define how things should get done as well as provide the basis for information that is or will be required by regulatory authorities. Documentation is necessary for employees to understand how work should be done. These documents should be used for training purposes. With proper training, employees can be held accountable for their job responsibilities. It is crucial to show employees how you expect the work to change.

Let's say for example, that your assessment of a workflow in operations revealed a missed step in required sanitation. You need to first determine if it is required already, but not being followed, or if it was never required. You can ask, but you are likely to get different answers from different people.

- If no documentation exists today (worst case), you can't tell if they were supposed to be doing it. The absence of documentation

TABLE A.1 How the Organization Deals With Tribal Knowledge Versus Process Documentation

How the Organization Deals With...	Tribal Knowledge	Process Documentation System
Work Process Knowledge	Owned by individuals	Individuals share knowledge so everyone owns it
Knowledge Collection	Informal and in individual's notes	Formally collected and retained in procedures
Task Performance	By each individual in the individual's best way	Everyone utilizes agreed-upon most efficient way
Challenges	Each individual determines how to address problems in a vacuum. Frequent use of "work-arounds."	Everyone works together to work to systemic solutions to problems, based on root cause analysis
New learning	New people learn by doing or depend on others	New people have full access to the body of knowledge contained in processes
Work Verifications	None formalized	Formalized, specified checkpoint list

shows that they don't know either. You will need to write documentation concerning the missed step. You will need to add the step to job descriptions and train managers and employees on the new expectation. In this scenario, your organization taps heavily into "Tribal Knowledge," which has some clear challenges. See the matrix (Table A.1) at the end of this section.

- If good documentation exists but does not include that step, a process change is needed. You will need to add it to the documentation, the job descriptions, and train managers and employees on the new expectation. This is easier than starting documentation from scratch but will still involve good attention to detail on your part.

- If good documentation exists today, and it includes that step (best-case), you will need to re-train. Make sure your training includes teaching the managers how to hold employees accountable for expectations and how to use existing documentation to do so.

The first litmus test as to whether your organization has a good process documentation system is to ask yourself if when you were put into your position there was good/adequate documentation to support the processes in your department.

- Did you get trained? Were there training manuals? Were they accurate?
- Can you look at the documents now if something comes up that you don't remember? Do you know how to find them? Is the information available to you accurate?
- Do you have a process manual for the whole organization? Is it current?
- Do you have a Policies Manual? Is it current?

If the answer is yes, you were fully trained and have great documentation. Be sure that it exists with the teams you are supporting.

If the answer is no, you saw none of this when you started, or you saw only some of these things, when you started, you should investigate further. You may not have seen them because your department is small. It is also possible that you have been in your role too long to know what they are doing now.

When you look further, the next step would be to see how widespread the absence of good documentation is. Find three to five positions in your organization where there are several people who do that work. Then, ask them about their training to see if there is good documentation. Most often, planned change does not get done because the organization is unable to thoroughly manage the details of the work.

In order for you to set up a good *Roadmap* for Food Safety, you will need an existing documentation process to work within. If you don't have one, you should be influencing the organization to set one up. That will take time. You can be doing your work in the meantime, but be sure you document the processes for the employees in the most effective way possible. Create your Roadmap so that the organization will want to follow, that is, because they see how it will help them and the company.

If you need to garner more support, Table A.1 shows the challenges inherent in "Tribal Knowledge."

CORPORATE COMMUNICATION SYSTEMS

Communication is often very ineffective across organizations. As a result, there are no strong ways for you to engage when you need to communicate information. Most often, they don't exist because people don't place a premium on the communication necessary to support change. Since effective communication is critical to your efforts, you will find that you and any committee you put in place to assist you will have to determine how to effectively communicate. It is of course, much easier for you to get your work done if the entire organization embraces and understands effective communication.

Here are a few key elements to set up in good communication systems.

- Regular meetings are needed. They should be effective, focused, and consistent. They should take place for leaders, at various levels, and for all departments and teams. They may be daily, weekly, monthly, or with some other degree of regularity. There should be a meeting leader who communicates about the meeting, publishes an agenda, and effectively runs the meeting. Meetings should have published minutes for all participants with assigned action points that have due dates for completion or reporting. An organization has an effective meeting system if you can roll out a change over the course of several weeks by having the meetings, and accurately disseminating the meetings' findings and action points. If this is the case, everyone in your organization is getting information on a regular basis.
  - ○ Meetings may be daily huddles.

- o Meetings may be weekly stand-ins, lasting 15 min and covering the news of the week.
- o Meetings for leaders and managers should be regular and at least monthly. They should include the review of progress on strategic initiatives, placing Food Safety on every agenda.
- o Meetings regarding strategy should be at least quarterly, adjusting the strategy where necessary.
- o Department meetings with all employees should be at least every other month.
- Effective electronic communications are key. Corporate update e-mails, intranet/social networking in closed groups, and electronic newsletters or company videos are all tools to put in place to support effective communication. Each form of communication should have an owner who strategically plans what is being shared with the employees, so that it supports what the organization is trying to do. Sometimes this rests in Human Resources (HR) or with an Executive Assistant for a key leader. Sometimes there is a designated person with this as his/her sole responsibility. Whether or not it is this person's only responsibility or it is added onto other responsibilities, it is a factor that affects how available and flexible the resource can be. If none of these roles exist, start one, or start influencing leaders to consider adding some.
- In-office communication might include posters, fliers, and handouts at meetings with key messages. These are easy for managers to do, but if you want them to support your work by adding this to their communications, you will have to ask them to do so. If they aren't used to doing this kind of communication, help them do it one time to carry your message. This will make it easier the next time you need help.
- Finally, managers must be able to communicate with employee teams as a group and one-on-one about positive and constructive things. If you see an absence of these skills around you, suggest training for managers on communication and influence.

Here are some ground rules for communication to share with your managers:

- Many changes are too confidential to share. However, the more transparency you can offer, the easier it will be for people to understand and receive the information.

- Involve everyone you can in the dialog to plan and make the change.
- Pre-sell the changes with everyone you can to get buy-in and support, and to understand concerns.
- Cover substantial change with each person affected in a one-on-one private meeting (new boss, new job, loss of an area of focus, substantial changes in focus, etc.).
- If change involves many people, have your announcements take place in a small window of time: simultaneously if possible, or within a short timespan if the nature of the change requires one-on-one private meetings.
- Successful change communication requires willingness to be repetitive with the message and have multiple touch points to ensure the changes happen as planned. This is where ongoing systems are needed.

JOB DESCRIPTIONS-BASED PERFORMANCE REVIEW SYSTEMS`

Job Descriptions and related key performance indicators are a way to define what is expected of a person regarding Food Safety. They will span objectives far beyond Food Safety. If you add Food Safety to this system as a way to outline expectations and hold people accountable (both of which are critical for substantiate change), the system must exist and be effective.

Many organizations have inadequate Job Descriptions or none at all and generic Performance Reviews. This type of HR management will dilute your efforts in Food Safety. You may find that you need to influence the implementation of the right type of performance management system so that you can effectively do what you need to do and be able to hold people within the organization accountable for their actions. You will have to in all likelihood influence the HR leader responsible for performance management. He or she may have another level of leadership to convince, so you can help them. Doing so will help them with their talent planning, talent development, and hiring/placement, in addition to Performance Management.

Here are some things that will help you with the conversation.

Consider these things when creating Job Descriptions:

- Jobs are made up of tasks. These are the things the *position* actually does, on a day-to-day basis. The things this position is responsible to complete or accomplish.
- Jobs exist to produce results. Usually, the results are outcomes that are measured and part of the *person's* regular performance achievement.
- Jobs can only be done well, with good completion of tasks and good fulfillment of the desired outcomes when the *person in the position* has the *skills* required of the job.

Therefore, the process to determine what *competencies* a *person* needs for a particular *position* is as follows:

1. Identify the process to be followed by the *person in the position*.
2. Identify the tasks that make up the process, and determine which exact tasks are the responsibility of the *person in the position*.
3. Identify the expected outcomes of the *person in the position*.
4. Determine which *skills* are needed by the *person in the position* to complete the tasks and produce the expected results.
5. Group the *skills* into related *competency clusters* to keep the number of skills manageable and to enable precise definition of what is needed.
6. Determine the criteria for mastery within each *competency cluster*, and the minimum requirements for the position. This can then be used in selecting the right *person for the position* and developing that *person* to be stronger in their *position*.

Fig. A.1 describes what needs to be addressed to develop a good job description.

Next, you connect the Job Description with the Performance Management Documents so that participants can be held fully accountable for their required job functions and expected results.

PROCESS CHANGE, A MODEL...

Any improvement in Food Safety will require process change. While this is dealt with in the main segments of the book, the

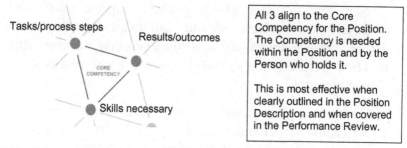

Tasks/process steps

Results/outcomes

CORE
COMPETENCY

Skills necessary

All 3 align to the Core
Competency for the Position.
The Competency is needed
within the Position and by the
Person who holds it.

This is most effective when
clearly outlined in the Position
Description and when covered
in the Performance Review.

FIGURE A.1   Model for alignment of Job Description.

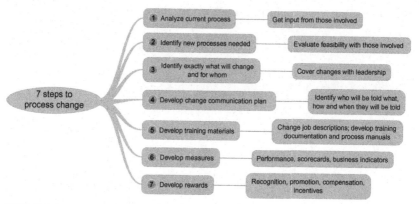

7 steps to
process change

1 Analyze current process — Get input from those involved

2 Identify new processes needed — Evaluate feasibility with those involved

3 Identify exactly what will change
and for whom — Cover changes with leadership

4 Develop change communication plan — Identify who will be told what,
how and when they will be told

5 Develop training materials — Change job descriptions; develop training
documentation and process manuals

6 Develop measures — Performance, scorecards, business indicators

7 Develop rewards — Recognition, promotion, compensation,
incentives

FIGURE A.2   A model for process change.

following diagram shows you how to move forward. Note the presence of so many of the things we talked about. Also note the need for the systems in process, change communication, and Job Description-related performance management (Fig. A.2).

- Steps 1 and 5 rely on the existence of a process documentation system.
- You will be responsible for identifying what is needed in new processes (Step 2) and in determining what change that will drive (Step 3).
- Then, once you know that, you will need to drive Step 4, change communication
  - Step 4 will rely on the existence of communication systems in order to operationalize your plan.

- o Note that this step also requires an update of the Job Description, which should automatically drive the Performance Review and how this person is held accountable.
- o The Job Description should also include the results expected and measured.

Following this process and ensuring these systems are established will allow for better accountability for the changes, supporting the culture change and obtaining the commitment.

The aforementioned information can be used by the Food Safety Professional to help them effectively do their job and in turn protect a company's consumer, customer, and brand.

Index

Note: Page numbers followed by "*t*" refer to tables.

Printed in the United States
By Bookmasters